Board Review Series

Embryology
2nd Edition

W9-AVN-177

Board Review Series

Embryology

2nd edition

Ronald W. Dudek, Ph.D.
Professor of Anatomy and Cell Biology
East Carolina University School of Medicine
Greenville, North Carolina

James D. Fix, Ph.D.
Professor Emeritus of Anatomy
Marshall University
School of Medicine
Huntington, West Virginia

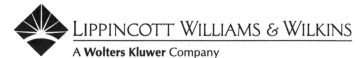

LIPPINCOTT WILLIAMS & WILKINS
A **Wolters Kluwer** Company
Philadelphia • Baltimore • New York • London
Buenos Aires • Hong Kong • Sydney • Tokyo

Editor: Elizabeth A. Nieginski
Managing Editor: Marette D. Magargle-Smith
Marketing Manager: Jennifer Conrad
Development Editor: Linda Weinerman

Copyright © 1998 Lippincott Williams & Wilkins

351 West Camden Street
Baltimore, Maryland 21201-2436 USA

Rose Tree Corporate Center
1400 North Providence Road
Building II, Suite 5025
Media, Pennsylvania 19063-2043 USA

All rights reserved. This book is protected by copyright. No part of this book may be reproduced in any form or by any means, including photocopying, or utilized by any information storage and retrieval system without written permission from the copyright owner.

The publisher is not responsible (as a matter of product liability, negligence or otherwise) for any injury resulting from any material contained herein. This publication contains information relating to general principles of medical care which should not be construed as specific instructions for individual patients. Manufacturers' product information and package inserts should be reviewed for current information, including contraindications, dosages and precautions.

Printed in the United States of America
First Edition,

Library of Congress Cataloging-in-Publication Data

Dudek, Ronald W., 1950–
    Embryology / Ronald W. Dudek, James D. Fix. —2nd ed.
        p.   cm. — (Board review series)
    Fix's name appears first on earlier ed.
    Includes bibliographical references and index.
    ISBN 0–683–30272–8
    1. Embryology, Human—Outlines, syllabi, etc. 2. Embryology,
Human—Examinations, questions, etc. I. Fix, James D., II. Title. III. Series.
    [DNLM: 1. Embryology outlines. 2. Embryology examination
Questions. QS 18.2 D845e 1998]
QM601.F68   1998
612.6'4'0076—dc21
DNLM/DLC
for Library of Congress   98–22361
                                                                                                              CIP

The publishers have made every effort to trace the copyright holders for borrowed material. If they have inadvertently overlooked any, they will be pleased to make the necessary arrangements at the first opportunity.

To purchase additional copies of this book, call our customer service department at **(800) 638-0672** or fax orders to **(800) 447-8438.** For other book services, including chapter reprints and large quantity sales, ask for the Special Sales department.

Canadian customers should call **(800) 665-1148,** or fax **(800) 665-0103.** For all other calls originating outside of the United States, please call **(410) 528-4223** or fax us at **(410) 528-8550.**

Visit Williams & Wilkins on the Internet: **http://www.wwilkins.com** or contact our customer service department at **custserv@wwilkins.com**. Williams & Wilkins customer service representatives are available from 8:30 am to 6:00 pm, EST, Monday through Friday, for telephone access.

                                                                                                              99 00
                                                                              2 3 4 5 6 7 8 9 10

Dedication

To Connor, Sean, and Katherine

Contents

Preface

The second edition of *BRS Embryology* has afforded us the opportunity to fine-tune a work that was already a highly rated course review book as well as an excellent review for the USMLE Step 1.

We have expanded the Cardiovascular System and Nervous System chapters (both text and illustrations) to include many more congenital malformations. (These systems are always well-represented on the USMLE.) We have rewritten the chapters on the Skeletal System and Muscular System in a much more clear and concise manner. And we have added two new chapters, Upper Limb Development and Lower Limb Development. The various aspects of limb development are detailed, with special emphasis on bone development and its importance in interpreting limb radiographs of newborns and children.

We hope that students will continue to find *BRS Embryology* a clear and thorough review of embryology. After taking USMLE Step 1, we invite our readers to e-mail Dr. Dudek at **dudek@brody.med.ecu.edu** to convey any comments or suggestions, or to indicate any area that was particularly represented on the USMLE.

Ronald W. Dudek

James D. Fix

1
Prefertilization Events

I. Sexual Reproduction
– occurs when female and male gametes (oocyte and spermatozoon, respectively) unite at fertilization.

A. Gametes
– are direct descendants of **primordial germ cells**, which are first observed in **the wall of the yolk sac** at week 4 of embryonic development and subsequently migrate into the future gonad region.
– are produced by **gametogenesis** (**oogenesis** in the female and **spermatogenesis** in the male).

B. Gametogenesis
– employs a specialized process of cell division, **meiosis**, which uniquely distributes chromosomes among gametes.

II. Chromosomes

A. General structure (Figure 1-1)

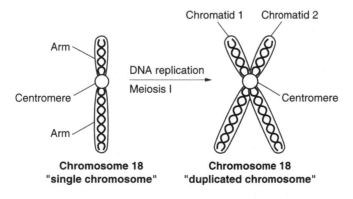

Figure 1-1. A schematic diagram of chromosome 18 shown in its "single chromosome" state and "duplicated chromosome" state, which is formed by DNA replication during meiosis I. It is important to understand that both the "single chromosome" state and "duplicated chromosome" state will be counted as one chromosome 18. As long as the additional DNA in the "duplicated chromosome" is bound at the centromere, the structure will be counted as one chromosome 18 even though it has twice the amount of DNA.

– A single chromosome consists of two characteristic regions called **arms**, which are separated by a **centromere**.

– During meiosis I, **single chromosomes** undergo DNA replication, which essentially duplicates the arms. This forms **duplicated chromosomes**, which consist of two sister **chromatids** attached at the centromere.

B. Ploidy and "N" number

– Cells can be designated by their number of chromosomes and amount of DNA, as shown in Table 1-1.

1. Definitions

a. Ploidy refers to **the number of chromosomes** in a cell.

b. The **"N" number** refers to the **amount of DNA** in a cell.

2. Normal somatic cells and primordial germ cells

– contain **46 single chromosomes** and **2N amount of DNA**; the chromosomes occur in **23 homologous pairs**; one member (homologue) of each pair is of maternal origin and the other is of paternal origin.

– The term "diploid" is classically used to refer to a cell containing 46 single chromosomes.

a. Pairs 1 to 22 are **autosomal (non-sex) pairs**.

b. Pair 23 consists of the **sex chromosomes** (XX for a female or XY for a male).

3. Gametes

– contain **23 single chromosomes** (22 autosomes and 1 sex chromosome) and **1N amount of DNA**.

– The term "haploid" is classically used to refer to a cell containing 23 single chromosomes.

a. Female gametes contain only the X sex chromosome.

Table 1-1. Cell Type and Designation of Number of Chromosomes and Amount of DNA

Cell Type	(# of chromosomes, amt. of DNA)
Primordial germ cells Oogonia Spermatogonia (Type A and B) Zygote Blastomeres All normal somatic cells	(46, 2N)
Primary oocyte Primary spermatocyte	(46, 4N)
Secondary oocyte Secondary spermatocyte	(23, 2N)
Mature oocyte (ovum) Spermatid Sperm	(23, 1N)

b. Male gametes contain either the X or Y sex chromosome; therefore, the male gamete determines the genetic sex of the individual.

C. The X chromosome

– A normal female somatic cell contains **two X chromosomes (XX)**.

– The female cell has evolved a mechanism for permanent **inactivation** of one of the X chromosomes, which occurs during week 1 of embryonic development.

1. The choice of which X chromosome (maternal or paternal) is inactivated seems to be random.

2. The inactivated X chromosome, which can be seen by light microscopy near the nuclear membrane, is called the **Barr body**.

D. The Y chromosome

– A normal male somatic cell contains **one X chromosome** and **one Y chromosome (XY)**.

– can be stained with certain fluorescent dyes and seen as a bright spot in the nucleus.

III. Meiosis (Figure 1-2)

A. Definition

– Meiosis is a specialized process of cell division that occurs only in the production of gametes. It consists of two divisions that result in the formation of four gametes, each containing half the number of chromosomes (23 single chromosomes) and half the amount of DNA (1N) found in normal somatic cells (46 single chromosomes, 2N).

B. Important events during meiosis

1. Meiosis I

a. Synapsis: pairing of 46 homologous duplicated chromosomes.

b. Crossing over: large segments of DNA are exchanged.

c. Alignment: 46 homologous duplicated chromosomes align at the metaphase plate.

d. Disjunction: 46 homologous duplicated chromosomes separate from each other; **centromeres do not split.**

e. Cell division: two secondary gametocytes (23 duplicated chromosomes, 2N) are formed.

2. Meiosis II

a. Synapsis: absent

b. Crossing over: absent

c. Alignment: 23 duplicated chromosomes align at the metaphase plate.

d. Disjunction: 23 duplicated chromosomes separate to form 23 single chromosomes; **centromeres split.**

e. Cell division: four gametes (23 single chromosomes, 1N) are formed.

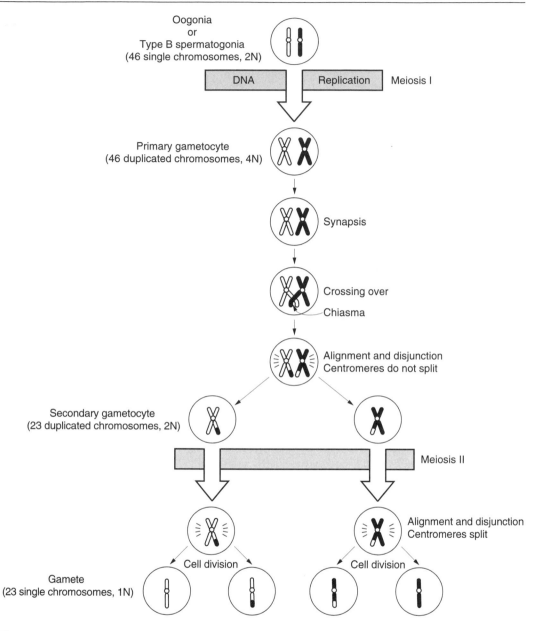

Figure 1-2. Schematic representation of meiosis I and meiosis II, emphasizing the changes in chromosome number and amount of DNA that occur during gametogenesis (either oogenesis or spermatogenesis). Only one pair of homologous chromosomes is shown (white = maternal origin and black = paternal origin). The point at which DNA crosses over is called the chiasma. Segments of DNA are exchanged, thereby introducing genetic variability to the gametes.

IV. Consideration of Female Events

A. Oogenesis: Formation of the female gamete

1. **Primordial germ cells** arrive in the gonad of a genetic female (ovary) at **week 4** and differentiate into **oogonia**, which populate the ovary through mitotic division.

2. Oogonia give rise to **primary oocytes** by undergoing DNA replication.

3. All primary oocytes are formed by **month 5 of fetal life**; no oogonia are present at birth.

4. Primary oocytes remain dormant in **prophase (dictyotene) of meiosis I** from month 5 of fetal life until puberty. After puberty, from 5 to 15 primary oocytes will begin maturation with each ovarian cycle, with usually only one reaching full maturity in each cycle.

   a. After puberty, a primary oocyte completes meiosis I to form two daughter cells: the **secondary oocyte** and the **first polar body**, which degenerates.

   b. The secondary oocyte enters meiosis II. When the chromosomes align at the metaphase plate, ovulation occurs. After this point, oogenesis is completed in the uterine tube, where fertilization occurs.

   c. The secondary oocyte remains **arrested in metaphase of meiosis II** until fertilization occurs.

   d. At fertilization, the secondary oocyte will complete meiosis II to form a **mature oocyte** and a **second polar body**.

B. Approximate number of oocytes

1. **Primary oocytes**: At month 5 of fetal life, 7 million are present. At birth, 2 million are present (5 million have degenerated). At puberty, 40,000 are present (1.96 million more have degenerated).

2. **Secondary oocytes**: 12 are ovulated per year, up to 480 over the entire reproductive life of the woman (40 years x 12 secondary oocytes per year = 480). This number (480) is obviously oversimplified since it is **reduced** in women who take birth control pills (which prevent ovulation), in women who become pregnant (ovulation stops during pregnancy), and in women who may have anovulatory cycles.

V. Consideration of Male Events

A. Spermatogenesis: Formation of the male gamete

– Classically, spermatogenesis is divided into three phases: spermatocytogenesis, meiosis, and spermiogenesis.

1. **Primordial germ cells** arrive in the gonad of a genetic male (testes) at **week 4** and remain **dormant until puberty**.

2. At puberty, primordial germ cells differentiate into **Type A spermatogonia**, which undergo mitosis to provide a continuous supply of stem cells throughout the reproductive life of the male (spermatocytogenesis). Some Type A spermatogonia differentiate into **Type B spermatogonia**.

   a. Type B spermatogonia give rise to **primary spermatocytes** by undergoing DNA replication.

   b. Primary spermatocytes complete meiosis I to form **two secondary spermatocytes**.

c. The two secondary spermatocytes complete meiosis II to form four **spermatids**.

d. Spermatids undergo a series of **morphological** changes that result in the formation of spermatozoa (spermiogenesis). These changes include formation of the acrosome, condensation of the nucleus, and formation of head, neck, and tail. The total time of sperm formation (from spermatogonia to spermatozoa) is about 64 days.

B. Capacitation of sperm
   – is a reversible process whereby freshly ejaculated sperm develop the capacity to fertilize a secondary oocyte.
   – normally occurs in the female reproductive tract and takes 7 hours.
   – involves the following:

1. Unmasking of glycosyltransferases on the sperm cell membrane

2. Removal of surface-coating proteins derived from seminal fluid

VI. Clinical Considerations

A. Offspring of older women

1. Prolonged dormancy of primary oocytes may be the reason for the high incidence of chromosomal abnormalities in offspring of older women.
   – Since all primary oocytes are formed by month 5 of fetal life, a female infant is born with her entire supply of gametes.
   – Primary oocytes remain dormant until ovulation; those ovulated late in the woman's reproductive life may have been dormant for as long as 40 years.

2. The incidence of **trisomy 21 (Down syndrome)** increases with advanced age of the mother.

B. Offspring of older men
   – An increased incidence of **achondroplasia** (a congenital skeletal anomaly characterized by retarded bone growth) is associated with advanced paternal age.

C. Male fertility
   – depends on the number and motility of sperm.

1. The average volume of semen in a normal, fertile male ejaculate is 3.5 ml, with a concentration of about 100 million sperm/ml of semen. Sterile males produce less than 20 million sperm/ml of semen.

2. Normally up to 10% of sperm in an ejaculate may be grossly deformed (two heads or two tails), but these sperm probably do not fertilize an oocyte owing to their lack of motility.

D. Female fertility and hormonal contraception

1. Oral contraceptives
   – contain low levels of **estrogen** and the progesterone analog **progestin**.

- prevent ovulation by maintaining elevated levels of estrogen and progestin, which inhibit the release of follicle-stimulating hormone (FSH) and luteinizing hormone (LH).
- can be used for "morning-after" contraception: 2 pills are taken up to 72 hours after intercourse followed by 2 pills 12 hours later; will prevent 75% of pregnancies.

2. Medroxyprogesterone acetate (Depo-Provera)
- is a long-acting alternative to oral contraceptives.
- can be injected **intramuscularly** and will prevent ovulation **for 2–3 months**.

3. Levonorgestrel (Norplant)
- offers an even longer-acting alternative; capsules containing levonorgestrel can be implanted **subdermally** and will prevent ovulation **for 1–5 years**.

4. The estimated chance of pregnancy (fertility) in the days surrounding ovulation is shown in Table 1-2.

E. Nondisjunction

1. In normal meiosis I and meiosis II, disjunction occurs (duplicated chromosomes align at the metaphase plate and separate from each other equivalently); as a result, gametes with 23 single chromosomes are produced.

2. If meiosis I or meiosis II proceeds abnormally, equivalent chromosome separation does not occur (nondisjunction); as a result, abnormal gametes with 24 single chromosomes and 22 single chromosomes are produced.

a. Fertilization between a normal gamete and an abnormal gamete with 24 single chromosomes will produce an individual with 47 single chromosomes (23 + 24 = 47), known as **trisomy**.

b. Fertilization between a normal gamete and an abnormal gamete with 22 single chromosomes will produce an individual with 45 single chromosomes (23 + 22 = 45), known as **monosomy**.

Table 1-2. Chance of Pregnancy in the Days Surrounding Ovulation

5 days before ovulation—10%
4 days before ovulation—16%
3 days before ovulation—14%
2 days before ovulation—27%
1 days before ovulation—31%
Day of ovulation—33%
Day after ovulation—0%

Review Test

Directions: Each of the numbered items or incomplete statements in this section is followed by answers or by completions of the statement. Select the **one** lettered answer or completion that is **best** in each case.

1. Which of the following is a major characteristic of meiosis I?

(A) Splitting of the centromere
(B) Pairing of homologous chromosomes
(C) Reducing the amount of DNA to 1N
(D) Achieving the diploid number of chromosomes
(E) Producing primordial germ cells

2. A normal somatic cell contains a total of 46 chromosomes. What is the normal complement of chromosomes found in a sperm?

(A) 22 autosomes plus a sex chromosome
(B) 23 autosomes plus a sex chromosome
(C) 22 autosomes
(D) 23 autosomes
(E) 23 paired autosomes

3. Which of the following describes the number of chromosomes and amount of DNA in a gamete?

(A) 46 chromosomes, 1N
(B) 46 chromosomes, 2N
(C) 23 chromosomes, 1N
(D) 23 chromosomes, 2N
(E) 23 chromosomes, 4N

4. Which of the following chromosome compositions in a sperm normally results in the production of a genetic female if fertilization occurs?

(A) 23 homologous pairs of chromosomes
(B) 22 homologous pairs of chromosomes
(C) 23 autosomes plus an X chromosome
(D) 22 autosomes plus a Y chromosome
(E) 22 autosomes plus an X chromosome

5. In the process of meiosis, DNA replication of each chromosome occurs, thereby forming a structure consisting of two sister chromatids attached to a single centromere. What is this structure?

(A) A duplicated chromosome
(B) Two chromosomes
(C) A synapsed chromosome
(D) A crossover chromosome
(E) A homologous pair

6. All primary oocytes are formed by

(A) week 4 of embryonic life
(B) month 5 of fetal life
(C) birth
(D) month 5 of infancy
(E) puberty

7. When does formation of primary spermatocytes begin?

(A) During week 4 of embryonic life
(B) During month 5 of fetal life
(C) At birth
(D) During month 5 of infancy
(E) At puberty

8. In the production of female gametes, which of the following cells can remain dormant for 12 to 40 years?

(A) Primordial germ cell
(B) Primary oocyte
(C) Secondary oocyte
(D) First polar body
(E) Second polar body

9. In the production of male gametes, which of the following cells remains dormant for 12 years?

(A) Primordial germ cell
(B) Primary spermatocyte
(C) Secondary spermatocyte
(D) Spermatid
(E) Sperm

10. Approximately how many sperm will be ejaculated by a normal fertile male during sexual intercourse?

(A) 10 million
(B) 20 million
(C) 35 million
(D) 100 million
(E) 350 million

11. A young woman enters puberty with approximately 40,000 primary oocytes in her ovary. About how many of these primary oocytes will be ovulated over the entire reproductive life of the woman?

(A) 40,000
(B) 35,000
(C) 480
(D) 48
(E) 12

12. Fetal sex can be diagnosed by noting the presence or absence of the Barr body in cells obtained from the amniotic fluid. What is the etiology of the Barr body?

(A) Inactivation of both X chromosomes
(B) Inactivation of homologous chromosomes
(C) Inactivation of one Y chromosome
(D) Inactivation of one X chromosome
(E) Inactivation of one chromatid

13. How much DNA does a primary spermatocyte contain?

(A) 1N
(B) 2N
(C) 4N
(D) 6N
(E) 8N

14. During meiosis, pairing of homologous chromosomes occurs, which permits large segments of DNA to be exchanged. What is this latter process called?

(A) Synapsis
(B) Nondisjunction
(C) Alignment
(D) Crossing over
(E) Disjunction

Directions: Each group of items in this section consists of lettered options followed by a set of numbered items. For each item, select the **one** lettered option that is most closely associated with it. Each lettered option may be selected once, more than once, or not at all.

Questions 15–21

Match each of the following cells or conditions involved in gametogenesis with the appropriate number of chromosomes.

(A) 22 chromosomes
(B) 23 chromosomes
(C) 23 duplicated chromosomes
(D) 24 chromosomes
(E) 45 chromosomes
(F) 46 chromosomes
(G) 46 duplicated chromosomes
(H) 47 chromosomes

15. Primary gametocyte

16. Normal female gamete

17. Secondary gametocyte

18. Trisomy

19. Monosomy

20. Abnormal gamete involved in producing trisomy

21. Abnormal gamete involved in producing monosomy

Answers and Explanations

1–B. Pairing of homologous chromosomes (synapsis) is a unique event that occurs only during meiosis I in the production of gametes. Synapsis is necessary so that crossing over can occur.

2–A. A normal gamete (sperm in this case) contains 23 single chromosomes. These 23 chromosomes consist of 22 autosomes plus 1 sex chromosome.

3–C. Gametes contain 23 chromosomes and 1N amount of DNA, so that when two gametes fuse at fertilization, a zygote containing 46 chromosomes and 2N amount of DNA will be formed.

4–E. A sperm contains 22 autosomes and 1 sex chromosome. The sex chromosome in sperm may be either the X or Y chromosome. The sex chromosome in a secondary oocyte is only the X chromosome. If an X-bearing sperm fertilizes a secondary oocyte, a genetic female (XX) is produced. Therefore, sperm is the arbiter of sex determination.

5–A. The structure formed is a duplicated chromosome. DNA replication occurs so that the amount of DNA is doubled (2 x 2N = 4N). However, the chromatids remain attached to the centromere, forming a duplicated chromosome.

6–B. During early fetal life, oogonia undergo mitotic divisions to populate the developing ovary. All the oogonia subsequently give rise to primary oocytes by month 5 of fetal life; at birth no oogonia are present in the ovary. At birth, a female has her entire supply of primary oocytes to carry her through reproductive life.

7–E. At birth, a male has primordial germ cells in the testes that remain dormant until puberty, at which time they differentiate into Type A spermatogonia. At puberty, some Type A spermatogonia differentiate into Type B spermatogonia and give rise to primary spermatocytes by undergoing DNA replication.

8–B. Primary oocytes are formed by month 5 of fetal life and remain dormant until puberty when hormonal changes in the young woman stimulate the ovarian and menstrual cycles. From 5 to 15 oocytes will then begin maturation with each ovarian cycle throughout the woman's reproductive life.

9–A. Primordial germ cells migrate from the wall of the yolk sac during the week 4 of embryonic life and enter the gonad of a genetic male where they remain dormant until puberty (about age 12) when hormonal changes in the young man stimulate the production of sperm.

10–E. A normal fertile male will ejaculate about 3.5 ml of semen containing about 100 million sperm/ml (3.5 ml x 100 million = 350 million).

11–C. Over her reproductive life, a woman will ovulate approximately 480 oocytes. A woman will ovulate 12 primary oocytes per year provided that she is not using oral contraceptives, does not become pregnant, or does not have any anovulatory cycles. Assuming a 40-year reproductive period, 40 x 12 = 480.

12–D. The Barr body is formed from inactivation of one X chromosome in a female. All somatic cells of a normal female will contain two X chromosomes. The female has evolved a mechanism for permanent inactivation of one of the X chromosomes presumably because a double dose of X chromosome products would be lethal.

13–C. Type B spermatogonia give rise to primary spermatocytes by undergoing DNA replication, thereby doubling the amount of DNA (2 x 2N = 4N) within the cell.

14–D. Synapsis (pairing of homologous chromosomes) is a unique event that occurs only during meiosis I in the production of gametes. Synapsis is necessary so that crossing over, whereby large segments of DNA are exchanged, can occur.

15–G. A primary gametocyte contains 46 duplicated chromosomes due to DNA replication and the fact that all the DNA remains attached to the centromere.

16–B. A normal female gamete contains 23 chromosomes.

17–C. A secondary gametocyte contains 23 duplicated chromosomes after disjunction and cell division occur in meiosis I.

18–H. During meiosis, chromosomes align at the metaphase plate and then undergo disjunction; chromosomes go to opposite poles in preparation for cell division. If nondisjunction occurs, gametes with an extra chromosome may form and contribute to the production of an individual with 47 chromosomes, known as trisomy. Trisomy produces well-known clinical syndromes: trisomy 21 is Down syndrome, trisomy 18 is Edwards syndrome, and trisomy 13 is Patau syndrome.

19–E. If nondisjunction occurs during meiosis, gametes lacking one chromosome may form and contribute to the production of an individual with 45 chromosomes, known as monosomy. Monosomy X is known as Turner syndrome.

20–D. Gametes with an extra chromosome (24 chromosomes) may form because of nondisjunction during meiosis. These abnormal gametes contribute to the production of an individual with 47 chromosomes (trisomy) if joined with a normal gamete (23 chromosomes) at fertilization (24 + 23 = 47).

21–A. Gametes lacking one chromosome (22 chromosomes) may form because of nondisjunction during meiosis. These abnormal gametes contribute to the production of an individual with 45 chromosomes (monosomy) if joined with a normal gamete (23 chromosomes) at fertilization (22 + 23 = 45).

2

Week 1 of Human Development (Days 1–7)

I. Introduction
– The age of a developing conceptus can be measured either from the estimated day of fertilization (fertilization age) or from the day of the last normal menstrual period (LNMP age). In this book, age is presented as the fertilization age.

II. Three Phases of Fertilization
– Fertilization occurs in the **ampulla of the uterine tube**.

A. Phase 1: Sperm penetration of corona radiata
– is aided by action of sperm and uterine tube mucosal enzymes.

B. Phase 2: Sperm binding and penetration of zona pellucida

1. Sperm binding
– occurs through interaction of sperm glycosyltransferases and ZP3 receptors located on the zona pellucida.
– triggers the **acrosome reaction**, that is, the fusion of the outer acrosomal membrane and sperm cell membrane, resulting in the release of acrosomal enzymes.

2. Penetration of zona pellucida
– is aided by acrosomal enzymes, specifically **acrosin**.

a. Sperm contact with the cell membrane of a secondary oocyte triggers the **cortical reaction**, that is, the release of cortical granules (lysosomes) from the oocyte cytoplasm.

b. This reaction renders both the zona pellucida and oocyte membrane impermeable to other sperm.

C. Phase 3: Fusion of sperm and oocyte cell membranes

1. Both membranes bind and subsequently break down at the fusion area.

2. The entire sperm (except the cell membrane) enters the cytoplasm of secondary oocyte.

a. Sperm mitochondria and tail degenerate.

b. Sperm nucleus forms the **male pronucleus**.

3. Secondary oocyte completes meiosis II, forming a mature ovum and second polar body.

   – Nucleus of mature ovum is the **female pronucleus**.

4. Male and female pronuclei fuse, thereby forming a **zygote** (a new cell whose genotype is an intermingling of maternal and paternal chromosomes).

III. Cleavage and Blastocyst Formation (Figure 2-1)

A. Cleavage

– is a series of **mitotic** divisions of the zygote.

1. Zygote cytoplasm is successively partitioned (cleaved) to form a **blastula** consisting of increasingly smaller **blastomeres** (2-cell, 4-cell, 8-cell, and so on).

   – Blastomeres are considered totipotent (capable of forming a complete embryo) up to the 4- to 8-cell stage (important when considering monozygotic twinning).

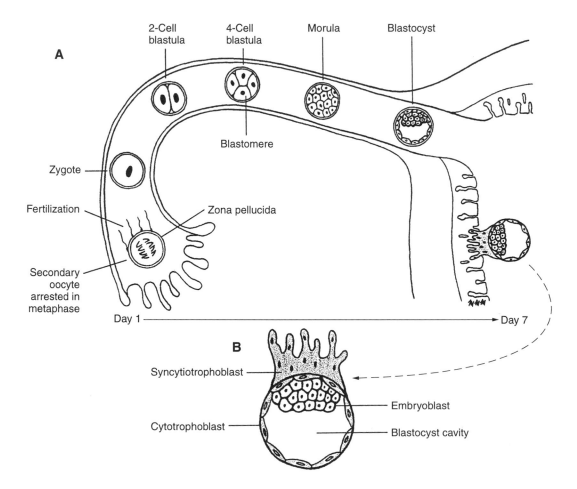

Figure 2-1. *(A)* The stages of human development during week 1. *(B)* A day 7 blastocyst. (Reprinted from Dudek RW: *High-Yield Embryology*. Baltimore, Williams & Wilkins, 1996, p. 5).

2. Blastomeres form a **morula** by undergoing **compaction**, that is, tight junctions are formed between the cells in the **outer cell mass**, thereby sealing off the **inner cell mass**.

  – **Uvomorulin**, a glycoprotein found on the surface of blastomeres, is involved in compaction.

B. Blastocyst formation

  – Fluid secreted within the morula forms the **blastocyst cavity**. The conceptus is now called a **blastocyst**.

1. The inner cell mass is now called the **embryoblast** (becomes the embryo).

2. The outer cell mass is now called the **trophoblast** (becomes fetal portion of the placenta).

C. Zona pellucida degeneration

  – occurs by day 4 after conception. The zona pellucida must degenerate for implantation to occur.

IV. Implantation (see Figure 2-1)

  – The blastocyst usually implants within the **posterior superior wall** of the uterus by **day 7** after fertilization. Implantation occurs in the **functional layer** of the endometrium during the **progestational (secretory) phase** of the menstrual cycle.
  – The trophoblast proliferates and differentiates into the **cytotrophoblast** and **syncytiotrophoblast**.
  – Failure of implantation may involve immune rejection (a graft-versus-host reaction) of the antigenic conceptus by the mother.

V. Clinical Considerations

A. Ectopic tubal pregnancy

  – is the **most common** type of ectopic pregnancy and occurs when the blastocyst implants abnormally within the uterine tube. Other ectopic implantation sites include the ovary, abdomen, internal ostium, and cervix.
  – is due to **delayed transport** through the uterine tube.
  – produces abdominal pain that may be confused with appendicitis; can lead to tubal rupture and hemorrhage, which can be circumvented by surgical removal of uterine tube and conceptus.

B. In vitro fertilization (IVF)

  – involves the retrieval of pre-ovulatory oocytes from the woman, in vitro fertilization by sperm, and culture to the 8- or 16-cell stage, followed by transfer to the uterus.

C. Teratocarcinoma

1. Spontaneous teratocarcinomas are **gonadal tumors** that contain both differentiated cell types and undifferentiated pluripotent stem cells called **embryonic carcinoma (EC) cells**.

2. Teratocarcinomas can be experimentally produced by implanting a blastocyst in an extrauterine site.

3. The ability of blastocysts to form teratocarcinomas suggests a relationship between the inner cell mass and EC cells.
   - This relationship has been confirmed by isolation of cell lines from blastocysts called embryonic stem (ES) cells, which have biochemical characteristics remarkably similar to EC cells.

Review Test

Directions: Each of the numbered items or incomplete statements in this section is followed by answers or by completions of the statement. Select the **one** lettered answer or completion that is **best** in each case.

1. A 20-year-old woman presents at the emergency department with severe abdominal pain on the right side with signs of internal bleeding. She indicated that she has been sexually active without contraception and missed her last menstrual period. Based on this information, which of the following disorders must be included as an option in the diagnosis?

(A) Ovarian cancer
(B) Appendicitis
(C) Normal pregnancy
(D) Ectopic tubal pregnancy
(E) Toxemia of pregnancy

2. When does a secondary oocyte complete its second meiotic division to become a mature ovum?

(A) At ovulation
(B) Before ovulation
(C) At fertilization
(D) At puberty
(E) Before birth

3. How soon after fertilization occurs within the uterine tube does the blastocyst begin implantation?

(A) Within minutes
(B) By 12 hours
(C) By day 1
(D) By day 2
(E) By day 7

4. Where does the blastocyst normally implant?

(A) Functional layer of the cervix
(B) Functional layer of the endometrium
(C) Basal layer of the endometrium
(D) Myometrium
(E) Perimetrium

5. Which of the following events is involved in cleavage of the zygote during week 1 of development?

(A) A series of meiotic divisions forming blastomeres
(B) Production of highly differentiated blastomeres
(C) An increased cytoplasmic content of blastomeres
(D) An increase in size of blastomeres
(E) A decrease in size of blastomeres

6. All of the following structures are necessary for blastocyst implantation EXCEPT

(A) endometrium in progestational phase
(B) zona pellucida
(C) syncytiotrophoblast
(D) cytotrophoblast
(E) functional layer of the endometrium

7. Which of the following is the origin of the mitochondrial DNA of all human adult cells?

(A) Paternal only
(B) Maternal only
(C) A combination of paternal and maternal
(D) Either paternal or maternal
(E) Unknown origin

8. Individual blastomeres were isolated from a blastula at the 4-cell stage. Each blastomere was cultured in vitro to the blastocyst stage and individually implanted into four pseudopregnant foster mothers. Which of the following would you expect to observe 9 months later?

(A) Birth of one baby
(B) Birth of four genetically different babies
(C) Birth of four genetically identical babies
(D) Birth of four grotesquely deformed babies
(E) No births

9. Embryonic carcinoma (EC) cells were isolated from a yellow-coated mouse with a teratocarcinoma. The EC cells were then micro-injected into the inner cell mass of a blastocyst isolated from a black-coated mouse. The blastocyst was subsequently implanted into the uterus of a white-coated foster mouse. Which of the following would be observed after full-term pregnancy?

(A) A yellow-coated offspring
(B) A black-coated offspring
(C) A white-coated offspring
(D) A yellow and black-coated offspring
(E) A yellow and white-coated offspring

Directions: Each group of items in this section consists of lettered options followed by a set of numbered items. For each item, select the **one** lettered option that is most closely associated with it. Each lettered option may be selected once, more than once, or not at all.

Questions 10–17

Match each of the cellular actions below with the most appropriate event.

(A) Fertilization
(B) Acrosome reaction
(C) Cortical reaction
(D) Compaction
(E) Cleavage
(F) Implantation

10. Release of acrosin

11. Causes zona pellucida impermeability

12. A series of mitotic divisions

13. Formation of tight junctions

14. Invasion by the syncytiotrophoblast

15. Completion of meiosis II

16. The glycoprotein uvomorulin

17. Graft-versus-host reaction

Answers and Explanations

1–D. Ectopic tubal pregnancy must always be an option in the diagnosis when a woman in her reproductive years presents with such symptoms. Ninety percent of ectopic implantations occur in the uterine tube. Ectopic tubal pregnancies result in rupture of the uterine tube and internal hemorrhage, which presents a major threat to the woman's life. The uterine tube and embryo must be surgically removed. The symptoms may sometimes be confused with appendicitis.

2–C. At ovulation, a secondary oocyte begins meiosis II, but this division is arrested at metaphase. The secondary oocyte will remain arrested in metaphase until a sperm penetrates it at fertilization. Therefore, the term "mature ovum" is somewhat of a misnomer, because it is a secondary oocyte that is fertilized and, once fertilized, the new diploid cell is known as a zygote. If fertilization does not occur, the secondary oocyte degenerates.

3–E. The blastocyst begins implantation by day 7 after fertilization.

4–B. The blastocyst implants in the functional layer of the uterine endometrium. The uterus is composed of the perimetrium, myometrium, and endometrium. Two layers are identified within the endometrium: (1) the functional layer, which is sloughed off at menstruation, and (2) the basal layer, which is retained at menstruation and serves as the source of regeneration of the functional layer. During the progestational phase of the menstrual cycle, the functional layer undergoes dramatic changes; uterine glands enlarge and vascularity increases in preparation for blastocyst implantation.

5–E. Cleavage is a series of mitotic divisions whereby the large amount of zygote cytoplasm is successively partitioned among the newly formed blastomeres. Although the number of blastomeres increases during cleavage, the size of individual blastomeres decreases until they resemble adult cells in size.

6–B. The zona pellucida must degenerate for implantation to occur. Early cleavage states of the blastula are surrounded by a zona pellucida, which prevents implantation in the uterine tube.

7–B. The mitochondrial DNA of all human adult cells is of maternal origin only. In human fertilization, the entire sperm enters the secondary oocyte cytoplasm. However, sperm mitochondria degenerate along with the sperm's tail. Therefore, only mitochondria present within the secondary oocyte (maternal) remain in the fertilized zygote.

8–C. This scenario would result in four genetically identical children. Blastomeres at the 4-cell to 8-cell stage are totipotent; that is, capable of forming an entire embryo. Since blastomeres arise by mitosis of the same cell (zygote), they are genetically identical. This phenomenon is important in explaining monozygotic (identical) twins. About 30% of monozygotic twins arise by early separation of blastomeres. The remaining 70% originate at the end of week 1 of development by a splitting of the inner cell mass.

9–D. This scenario would result in a yellow and black-coated offspring. Because EC cells and inner cell mass cells have very similar biochemical characteristics, they readily mix with each other and development proceeds unencumbered. Because the mixture contains cells with yellow-coat genotype and black-coat genotype, offspring with coats of two colors (yellow and black) will be produced. The offspring are known as mosaic mice.

10–B. The acrosome of sperm contains many different enzymes, such as hyaluronidase, acrosin, neuraminidase, corona-dispersing enzyme, and other trypsin-like enzymes. During the acrosome reaction, all these enzymes are released. Acrosin is specifically involved in digesting the zona pellucida.

11–C. Cortical granules, which are lysosomes within the cytoplasm of a secondary oocyte, release their contents (mucopolysaccharides and enzymes) as soon as the first sperm contacts the oocyte. The cortical granule contents not only coat the surface of the oocyte but also harden the zona pellucida, rendering it impermeable to other sperm. This blocks fertilization by more than one sperm.

12–E. After fertilization, the zygote undergoes a series of mitotic divisions called cleavage.

13–D. During cleavage, blastomeres are loosely arranged within the zona pellucida. Subsequently, the outer cells form tight junctions, thereby compacting the blastomeres and differentiating the outer cell mass from the inner cell mass.

14–F. Implantation begins by day 7 after fertilization as the syncytiotrophoblast begins invading the uterine endometrium.

15–A. The secondary oocyte will complete meiosis II only if fertilization occurs.

16–D. When tight junctions form during compaction, a glycoprotein called uvomorulin, located on the blastomere surface, is involved in the cell-to-cell attachments.

17–F. By day 7 after fertilization, the blastocyst (graft), with its unique genotype, begins to implant into the endometrium of the mother (host). Therefore, the mother is presented with antigenically different cells that she must tolerate if pregnancy is to continue.

3

Week 2 of Human Development (Days 8–14)

I. Further Development of the Embryoblast (Figure 3-1)

– The embryoblast differentiates into two distinct cellular layers: the dorsal **epiblast** layer (columnar cells) and the ventral **hypoblast** layer (cuboidal cells).

A. The epiblast and hypoblast form a flat, ovoid-shaped disk known as the **bilaminar embryonic disk**.

B. Clefts develop within the epiblast and coalesce to form the **amniotic cavity**.

C. Hypoblast cells begin to migrate and line the inner surface of the cytotrophoblast, forming the **exocoelomic membrane,** which delimits a space called the **exocoelomic cavity** (or **primitive yolk sac**). This space is later called the **definitive yolk sac** when a portion of the exocoelomic cavity is pinched off as an **exocoelomic cyst**.

D. At the future site of the mouth, hypoblast cells become columnar-shaped and fuse with epiblast cells to form a circular, midline thickening called the **prochordal plate**.

II. Further Development of the Trophoblast

A. Syncytiotrophoblast

– is the outer multinucleated zone of the trophoblast where no mitosis occurs.
– arises from the cytotrophoblast.
– continues invasion of the endometrial stroma, thereby eroding endometrial blood vessels and endometrial glands.

1. Lacunae form within the syncytiotrophoblast and become filled with nutritive maternal blood and glandular secretions. Endometrial stromal cells (**decidual cells**) at the site of implantation become filled with glycogen and lipids and also supply nutrients to the embryoblast.

a. Isolated lacunae fuse to form a **lacunar network**.

b. Maternal blood flows in and out of the lacunar network, thus establishing early **uteroplacental circulation**.

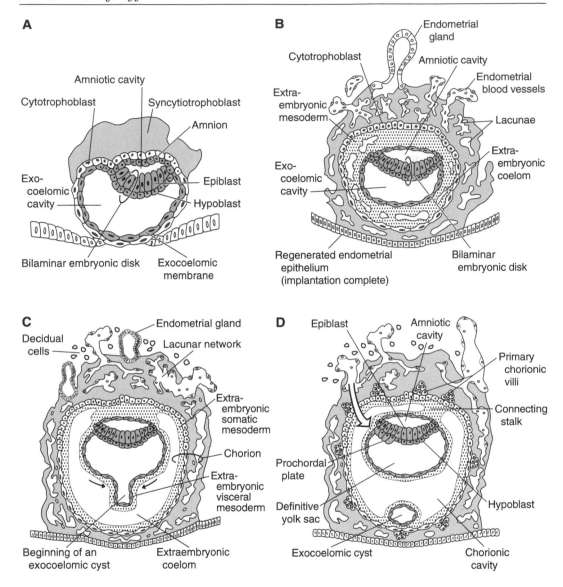

Figure 3-1. *(A)* Day 8 blastocyst is shown partially implanted into the endometrium. Extraembryonic mesoderm (EEM) has not formed yet. *(B)* Day 12 blastocyst is shown completely implanted within the endometrium, and epithelium has regenerated. This type of implantation is known as interstitial implantation. EEM begins to form. *(C)* Day 13 blastocyst. A lacunar network forms, establishing an early uteroplacental circulation. An exocoelomic cyst begins to pinch off *(small arrows). (D)* Day 14 blastocyst. The embryoblast can be described as two balloons (amniotic cavity and yolk sac) pressed together at the bilaminar embryonic disk. The curved open arrow indicates that the embryoblast receives maternal nutrients via diffusion.

2. Although a primitive circulation is established between the uterus and future placenta, the embryoblast receives its nutrition via diffusion only at this time.

B. Cytotrophoblast

– is mitotically active.

1. New cytotrophoblastic cells migrate into the syncytiotrophoblast, thereby fueling its growth.

2. New cytotrophoblastic cells produce local mounds called **primary chorionic villi** that bulge into the surrounding syncytiotrophoblast.

III. Development of Extraembryonic Mesoderm

A. The extraembryonic mesoderm develops from the epiblast and consists of loosely arranged cells.

B. This layer fills the space between the exocoelomic membrane and the cytotrophoblast.

C. Large spaces develop in the extraembryonic mesoderm and coalesce to form the **extraembryonic coelom**.

D. The extraembryonic coelom divides the extraembryonic mesoderm into the **extraembryonic somatic mesoderm** and **extraembryonic visceral mesoderm**.

   1. Extraembryonic somatic mesoderm lines the trophoblast, forms the connecting stalk, and covers the amnion.

   2. Extraembryonic visceral mesoderm covers the yolk sac.

E. Extraembryonic somatic mesoderm, cytotrophoblast, and syncytiotrophoblast constitute the **chorion**.

F. The extraembryonic coelom is now called the **chorionic cavity**.

G. The embryoblast is suspended by the **connecting stalk** within the chorionic cavity.

IV. Clinical Considerations

A. Human chorionic gonadotropin (hCG)
   – is a 57,000 MW glycoprotein with two subunits (alpha and beta) produced by the syncytiotrophoblast.
   – enters maternal blood circulation.
   – prevents degeneration of the corpus luteum.
   – stimulates production of progesterone in the corpus luteum and chorion, which sustains the placenta.
   – can be assayed in maternal blood at day 8 after fertilization and in maternal urine at day 10. This is the basis of early diagnosis of pregnancy.

B. Oncofetal antigens
   – are cell surface antigens that normally appear only on embryonic cells but for unknown reasons reexpress themselves in human malignant cells.
   – Monoclonal antibodies directed against specific oncofetal antigens provide an avenue for cancer therapy.
   1. Carcinoembryonic antigen (CEA) is associated with colorectal carcinoma.

   2. Alpha-fetoprotein is associated with hepatoma and germ cell tumors.

C. RU-486 (mifepristone)

- will initiate menstruation when taken within 8–10 weeks of the previous menses.
- If implantation of a conceptus has occurred, the conceptus will be sloughed along with the endometrium.
- is used in conjunction with prostaglandin and is 96% effective at terminating pregnancy.

Review Test

Directions: Each of the numbered items or incomplete statements in this section is followed by answers or by completions of the statement. Select the **one** lettered answer or completion that is **best** in each case.

1. Which of the following components plays the most active role in invading the endometrium during blastocyst implantation?

(A) Epiblast
(B) Syncytiotrophoblast
(C) Hypoblast
(D) Extraembryonic somatic mesoderm
(E) Extraembryonic visceral mesoderm

2. Between which two layers is the extraembryonic mesoderm located?

(A) Epiblast and hypoblast
(B) Syncytiotrophoblast and cytotrophoblast
(C) Syncytiotrophoblast and endometrium
(D) Exocoelomic membrane and syncytiotrophoblast
(E) Exocoelomic membrane and cytotrophoblast

3. During week 2 of development, the embryoblast receives its nutrients via

(A) diffusion
(B) osmosis
(C) reverse osmosis
(D) fetal capillaries
(E) yolk sac nourishment

4. The prochordal plate marks the site of the future

(A) umbilical cord
(B) heart
(C) mouth
(D) anus
(E) nose

5. Which of the following are components of the definitive chorion?

(A) Extraembryonic somatic mesoderm and epiblast
(B) Extraembryonic somatic mesoderm and cytotrophoblast
(C) Extraembryonic somatic mesoderm and syncytiotrophoblast
(D) Extraembryonic somatic mesoderm, cytotrophoblast, and syncytiotrophoblast
(E) Extraembryonic visceral mesoderm, cytotrophoblast, and syncytiotrophoblast

6. A 16-year-old girl presents on May 10 in obvious emotional distress. On questioning, she relates that on May 1 she experienced sexual intercourse for the first time, without any means of birth control. Most of her anxiety stems from her fear of pregnancy. What should the physician do to alleviate her fear?

(A) Prescribe diazepam and wait to see if she misses her next menstrual period
(B) Use ultrasonography to document pregnancy
(C) Order a laboratory assay for serum hCG
(D) Order a laboratory assay for serum progesterone
(E) Prescribe diethylstilbestrol ("morning-after pill")

7. Carcinoembryonic antigen (CEA) is an oncofetal antigen that is generally associated with which one of the following tumors?

(A) Hepatoma
(B) Germ cell tumor
(C) Squamous cell carcinoma
(D) Colorectal carcinoma
(E) Teratocarcinoma

Directions: The numbered items below correspond to lettered items in the figure. For each numbered item, select the **one** lettered option that is most closely associated with it. Each lettered option may be selected once, more than once, or not at all.

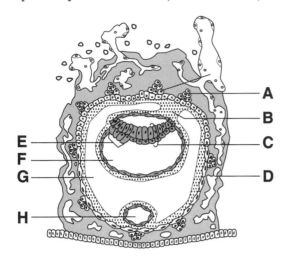

Questions 8–13

For each of the following statements or words concerning a 14-day-old blastocyst, select the most appropriate structure in the diagram.

8. Future site of the mouth

9. Forms definitive structures found in the adult

10. Chorion

11. Chorionic cavity

12. Primary chorionic villi

13. Connecting stalk

Answers and Explanations

1–B. The syncytiotrophoblast plays the most active role in invading the endometrium of the mother's uterus. During the invasion, endometrial blood vessels and endometrial glands are eroded and a lacunar network is formed.

2–E. The extraembryonic mesoderm is derived from the epiblast and is located between the exocoelomic membrane and the cytotrophoblast. The overall effect is to completely separate the embryoblast from the trophoblast, with the extraembryonic mesoderm serving as a conduit (connection) between them.

3–A. During week 2 of development, the embryoblast receives its nutrients from endometrial blood vessels, endometrial glands, and decidual cells via diffusion. Diffusion of nutrients does not pose a problem given the small size of the blastocyst during week 2. Although the beginnings of a uteroplacental circulation are established during week 2, no blood vessels have yet formed in the extraembryonic mesoderm to carry nutrients directly to the embryoblast (this occurs in week 3).

4–C. The prochordal plate is a circular, midline thickening of hypoblast cells that are firmly attached to the overlying epiblast cells. The plate will eventually develop into a membrane called the oropharyngeal membrane at the site of the future mouth. It is interesting to note that at this early stage of development, the cranial versus caudal region of the embryo is established by the prochordal plate. And since the prochordal plate is located in the midline, bilateral symmetry is also established.

5–D. The definitive chorion consists of three components: extraembryonic somatic mesoderm, cytotrophoblast, and syncytiotrophoblast. The chorion defines the chorionic cavity in which the embryoblast is suspended and is vital in the formation of the placenta.

6–C. Human chorionic gonadotropin (hCG) can be assayed in maternal serum at day 8 of development and in urine at day 10. If this teenager is pregnant, the blastocyst would be in week 2 of development (day 10). Laboratory assay of hCG in either the serum or urine can be completed; however, serum hCG might be more reliable. It is important to note that if she is pregnant, she will not miss a menstrual period until May 15, at which time the embryo will be entering week 3 of development.

7–D. Oncofetal antigens are normally expressed during embryonic development, remain unexpressed in normal adult cells, but reexpress on transformation to malignant neoplastic tissue. CEA is associated with colorectal carcinoma.

8–E. The prochordal plate indicates the site of the future mouth. At this early stage of development, the orientation of the embryo in the cranial versus caudal direction is established. The prochordal plate is a thickening of hypoblast cells that are firmly attached to the epiblast cells.

9–C. The bilaminar embryonic disk develops definitive adult structures after gastrulation occurs, as contrasted with the trophoblast, which is involved in placental formation.

10–D. The chorion consists of three layers; namely, extraembryonic somatic mesoderm, cytotrophoblast, and syncytiotrophoblast. The chorion is vital in the formation of the placenta.

11–G. The chorion forms the walls of the chorionic cavity in which the embryoblast is suspended by the connecting stalk. Note that the inner lining of the chorionic cavity is extraembryonic mesoderm.

12–A. The cytotrophoblast is mitotically active so that local mounds of cells (primary chorionic villi) form and bulge into the surrounding syncytiotrophoblast. As development continues, primary chorionic villi will form secondary chorionic villi and, finally, tertiary chorionic villi as part of placental formation.

13–B. The extraembryonic mesoderm can be thought of as initially forming in a continuous layer and then splitting as isolated cavities begin to appear everywhere except dorsally near the amniotic cavity and epiblast. When the isolated cavities coalesce, the extraembryonic coelom (or chorion cavity) and connecting stalk are formed.

4

Embryonic Period (Weeks 3–8)

I. General Considerations

A. All of the major organ systems begin to develop during the embryonic period [weeks 3–8 (days 15–56)].

B. Development of the cardiovascular system is essential because diffusion can no longer satisfy the nutritional needs of the embryo.

C. Folding of the embryo occurs.

    1. Craniocaudal folding is caused by the growth of the central nervous system (CNS) and the amnion.

    2. Lateral folding is caused by the growth of the somites, amnion, and other components of the lateral body wall.

    3. The craniocaudal folding and lateral folding change the shape of the embryo from a two-dimensional disk to a three-dimensional cylinder.

D. The embryo has a distinct human appearance by the end of week 8 of development.

    – The development of each individual organ system will be reviewed in upcoming chapters. However, it is important to realize that all organ systems develop simultaneously during the embryonic period.

II. Further Development of the Embryoblast

A. Gastrulation (Figure 4-1)

    – is the process that establishes the three definitive germ layers of embryo (**ectoderm, intraembryonic mesoderm,** and **endoderm**), thereby forming a **trilaminar embryonic disk** by day 21 of development. These three layers give rise to all the tissues and organs of the adult.

    – is first indicated by the formation of the **primitive streak**, caused by a proliferation of epiblast cells.

    1. The primitive streak consists of the **primitive groove, primitive node, and primitive pit.**

29

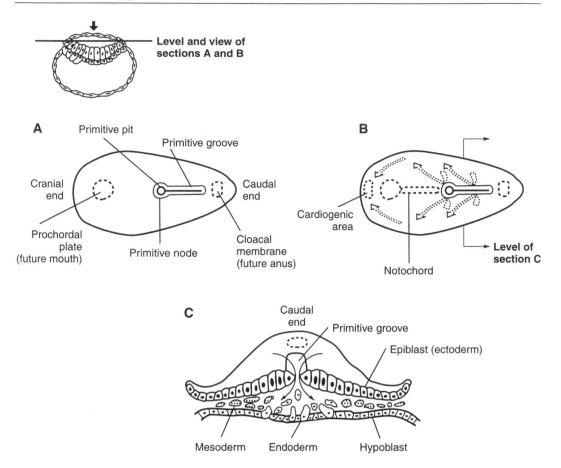

Figure 4-1. Schematic representation of gastrulation. Embryoblast in upper left is for orientation. *(A)* Dorsal view of the epiblast. *(B) Dotted arrows* show the migration of cells through the primitive streak during gastrulation. *(C)* Cross section showing the migration of cells that will form the intraembryonic mesoderm and displace the hypoblast to form endoderm. Epiblast cells begin to migrate to the primitive streak and invaginate into a space between the epiblast and hypoblast. Some of these migrating epiblast cells displace the hypoblast to form the definitive endoderm. The remainder of the epiblast cells migrate laterally, cranially, and along the midline to form the definitive intraembryonic mesoderm. After the formation of the endoderm and intraembryonic mesoderm, the epiblast is called the definitive ectoderm. (Reprinted from Dudek RW: *High-Yield Embryology.* Baltimore, Williams & Wilkins, 1996, p. 9.)

2. Located caudal to the primitive streak is the future site of the anus, known as the **cloacal membrane,** where epiblast and hypoblast cells are fused.

3. The ectoderm, intraembryonic mesoderm, and endoderm of the trilaminar embryonic disk are all derived from the epiblast.

4. The term *intraembryonic mesoderm* describes the germ layer that forms during week 3 (gastrulation) in contrast to the *extraembryonic mesoderm,* which formed during week 2. Intraembryonic mesoderm forms various tissues and organs found in the adult, whereas extraembryonic mesoderm is involved in placenta formation. Consequently, we will not use the term *intraembryonic* when discussing tissue and organ development of the adult in later chapters.

B. Changes involving intraembryonic mesoderm (Figure 4-2)

1. Paraxial mesoderm
   - is a thick plate of mesoderm on each side of the midline.
   - becomes organized into segments known as **somitomeres,** which form in a craniocaudal sequence.

   a. **Somitomeres 1–7** do not form somites but contribute mesoderm to the pharyngeal arches.

   b. The remaining somitomeres further condense in a craniocaudal sequence to form **42–44 pairs of somites**.

   c. The first pair of somites forms on day 20; new somites appear at a rate of 3/day.

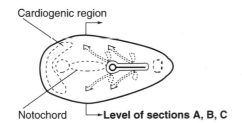

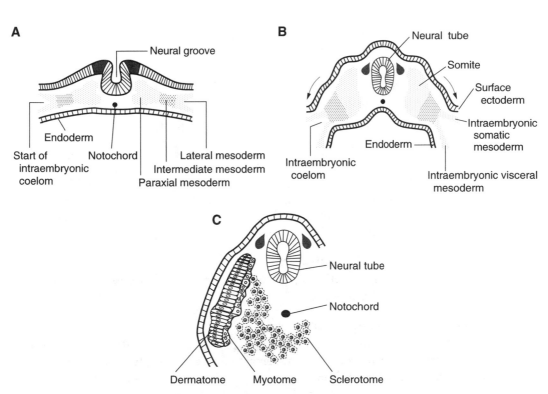

Figure 4-2. Schematic representation of changes involving intraembryonic mesoderm. Picture in upper left is for orientation. *(A)* Cross section at day 19. *(B)* Cross section at day 21, with *arrows* indicating lateral folding of the embryo. *(C)* Cross section showing differentiation of the somite.

d. The somites closest to the caudal end eventually disappear to give a final count of approximately **35 pairs of somites.**

e. The number of somites is one of the criteria for determining age of the embryo during this period.

f. Somites further differentiate into these components:

(1) Sclerotome (cartilage and bone component)

(2) Myotome (muscle component)

(3) Dermatome (dermis of skin component)

2. Intermediate mesoderm

– connects the paraxial mesoderm and lateral mesoderm.

– forms a longitudinal dorsal ridge known as the **urogenital ridge,** which is involved in the formation of the future **kidneys** and **gonads.**

3. Lateral mesoderm

– is a thin plate of mesoderm in which the **intraembryonic coelom** forms, dividing the lateral mesoderm into two layers:

a. Intraembryonic somatic mesoderm (also called somatopleure)

b. Intraembryonic visceral mesoderm (also called visceropleure or splanchnopleure)

4. Notochord

– is a solid cylinder of mesoderm extending in the midline of the trilaminar embryonic disk from the primitive node to the prochordal plate.

– is important for the following:

a. Induces the overlying ectoderm to differentiate into neuroectoderm to form the **neural plate.**

b. Induces the formation of the **vertebral bodies.**

c. Forms the **nucleus pulposus** of each intervertebral disk in a newborn.

5. Cardiogenic region

– is a horseshoe-shaped region of mesoderm located at the cranial end of the trilaminar embryonic disk, and is involved in the formation of the future **heart.**

C. Changes involving ectoderm

– Ectoderm is involved in the formation of the future **nervous system** and **epidermis of the skin.**

D. Changes involving endoderm

– Endoderm is involved in the formation of the future **digestive system,** future **respiratory system,** certain parts of the **urogenital system,** and **pharyngeal pouches.**

III. Angiogenesis (blood vessel formation)

A. In extraembryonic mesoderm

1. Angiogenesis occurs initially in extraembryonic visceral mesoderm **around the yolk sac** on day 17; by day 21, angiogenesis has occurred in extraembryonic somatic mesoderm around the connecting stalk to form the umbilical vessels and in secondary villi to form tertiary chorionic villi.

2. Extraembryonic mesoderm differentiates into **angioblasts,** which form clusters known as **angiogenic cell clusters.**

   a. Angioblasts located at the periphery of angiogenic cell clusters give rise to **endothelial cells.**

   b. Endothelial cells fuse with each other to form small blood vessels.

B. In intraembryonic mesoderm

   – Blood vessels form within the embryo by the same mechanism as in extraembryonic mesoderm.

C. Eventually blood vessels formed in the extraembryonic mesoderm will become continuous with blood vessels within the embryo, thereby establishing a blood vascular system between the embryo and the mother.

IV. Hematopoiesis (blood cell formation; Figure 4-3)

   – first occurs within the extraembryonic visceral mesoderm **around the yolk sac** during week 3 of development.

A. Angioblasts within the center of angiogenic cell clusters give rise to **primitive blood cells.**

B. Beginning at week 5, hematopoiesis is taken over by a sequence of embryonic organs: **liver, spleen, thymus,** and **bone marrow.**

C. Types of hemoglobin produced during hematopoeisis

   1. During the period of yolk sac hematopoieisis, the earliest **embryonic form** of hemoglobin, called **hemoglobin** $\zeta_2\epsilon_2$, is synthesized.

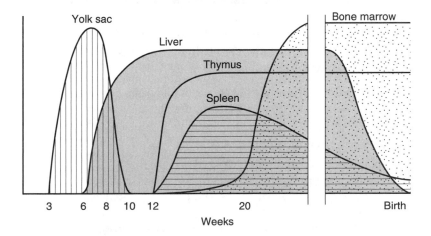

Figure 4-3. A schematic diagram showing the contribution of various organs to hematopoiesis during development.

2. During the period of liver hematopoiesis, the **fetal form** of hemoglobin, called **hemoglobin $\alpha_2\gamma_2$**, is synthesized. Hemoglobin $\alpha_2\gamma_2$ is the predominant form of hemoglobin during pregnancy because it has a higher affinity for oxygen than the adult form of hemoglobin (hemoglobin $\alpha_2\beta_2$) and thereby "pulls" oxygen from the maternal blood into fetal blood.

3. During the period of bone marrow hematopoiesis (about week 30), the **adult form** of hemoglobin, called **hemoglobin $\alpha_2\beta_2$**, is synthesized and gradually replaces hemoglobin $\alpha_2\gamma_2$.

D. The source of hematopoietic stem cells remains a mystery.

V. Clinical Considerations

A. Sacrococcygeal teratoma
– is a tumor that arises from remnants of the **primitive streak,** which normally degenerates and disappears.
– is derived from pluripotent cells of the primitive streak and often contains various types of tissue (e.g., bone, nerve, hair).
– occurs more commonly in female infants.
– usually becomes malignant during infancy and must be removed by age 6 months.

B. Chordoma
– is a tumor that arises from remnants of the **notochord.**
– may be found either intracranially or in the sacral region.
– occurs more commonly in men late in adult life (age 50).
– may be either benign or malignant.

C. Caudal dysplasia
– refers to a constellation of syndromes ranging from minor lesions of lower vertebrae to complete fusion of the lower limbs.
– is caused by **abnormal gastrulation,** in which the migration of mesoderm is disturbed.
– can be associated with various cranial anomalies:

1. **VATER,** which includes **Vertebral defects, Anal atresia, Tracheo-Esophageal fistula,** and **Renal defects**

2. **VACTERL,** which is similar to VATER but also includes **Cardiovascular defects** and **upper Limb defects**

D. Missed menstrual period
– is usually the **first indication of pregnancy.**
– Week 3 of embryonic development coincides with the first missed menstrual period. (Note that at this time the embryo has already undergone 2 weeks of development.)
– It is crucial that the woman become aware of a pregnancy as soon as possible because the embryonic period is a period of **high susceptibility to teratogens.**

E. Thalassemia syndromes

- are a heterogeneous group of genetic defects characterized by the lack of or decreased synthesis of either the α-globin chain (**α-thalassemia**) or β-globin chain (**β-thalassemia**) of hemoglobin $\alpha_2\beta_2$.
- **Hydrops fetalis** is the most severe form of α-thalassemia and causes severe pallor, generalized edema, massive hepatosplenomegaly, and invariably leads to intrauterine fetal death.
- **β-Thalassemia major** is the most severe form of β-thalassemia and causes a severe, transfusion-dependent anemia. It is most common in Mediterranean countries and parts of Africa and Southeast Asia.

VI. Summary of Germ Layer Derivatives (Table 4-1)

VII. Summary of Key Events in the Embryonic Period (Table 4-2)

Table 4-1. Summary of Germ Layer Derivatives

Ectoderm

Epidermis, hair, nails, sweat and sebaceous
  glands
Utricle, semicircular ducts, vestibular
  ganglion of CN VIII
Saccule, cochlear duct, spiral ganglion of
  CN VIII
Olfactory placodes, CN I
Ameloblasts
Adenohypophysis
Lens of eye
Anterior epithelium of the cornea
Acinar cells of parotid gland
Acinar cells of mammary gland
Epithelial lining of:
  Lower anal canal
  Distal part of male urethra
  External auditory meatus

Mesoderm

Muscle (smooth, cardiac, skeletal)
Extraocular muscles (preotic somites), ciliary
  muscle of eye, sclera, choroid, substantia
  propria of cornea, corneal endothelium
Muscles of tongue (occipital somites)
Pharyngeal arch muscles
Laryngeal cartilages
Connective tissue
Dermis of skin
Bone and cartilage
Dura mater
Endothelium of blood and lymph vessels
RBCs, WBCs, microglia, and Kupffer cells
Spleen
Kidney
Adrenal cortex
Testes and ovary

Endoderm

Hepatocytes
Principles and oxyphil of parathyroid
Thyroid follicular cells
Epithelial reticular cells of thymus
Acinar and islet cells of pancreas
Acinar cells of submandibular and sublingual
  glands
Epithelial lining of:
  GI tract
  Trachea, bronchi, lungs
  Biliary apparatus
  Urinary bladder, female urethra, most of
    male urethra
  Vagina
  Auditory tube, middle ear cavity
  Crypts of palatine tonsils

Neuroectoderm

All neurons within brain and spinal cord
  (CNS)
Retina, iris, ciliary body, optic nerve (CNS),
  optic chiasm, optic tract, dilator and
  sphincter muscles
Astrocytes, oligodendrocytes,
  ependymocytes, tanycytes, choroid plexus
  cells
Neurohypophysis
Pineal gland

Neural crest

Ganglia (dorsal root, cranial, autonomic)
Schwann cells
Odontoblasts
Pia and arachnoid
Chromaffin cells (adrenal medulla)
C cells of thyroid
Melanocytes
Aorticopulmonary septum
Pharyngeal arch skeletal components
Bones of neurocranium

CN = cranial nerve; *CNS* = central nervous system; *GI* = gastrointestinal; *RBCs* = red blood cells; *WBCs* =
white blood cells

Table 4-2. Summary of Key Events in the Embryonic Period

Week	Key Events	Appearance	Actual Size
3	Primitive streak appears Notochord appears Angiogenesis in yolk sac Gastrulation occurs Cranial neural folds elevated Early somites form	Day 21	3 mm
4	Neural tube forms Rostral/caudal neuropores close Otic/lens placode present Head and tail folding begins Lateral folding begins Upper/lower limb buds present Pharyngeal arches appear Heart is distinct	Day 28	5 mm
5	Upper limb is paddle-shaped Optic cup is present Hand plate forms Lower limb is paddle-shaped	Day 35	9 mm
6	Foot plate forms Auricular hillocks appear Digital rays appear in hand plate Cerebral vesicles prominent	Day 42	12 mm
7	Digital rays appear in foot plate Notches in hand plate form Both limbs extend ventrally Elbow region is apparent Notches in foot plate form	Day 48	15 mm
8	Fingers are formed Head is rounded Umbilical herniation distinct Toes are formed Tail disappears Distinct human appearance	Day 56	27 mm

Review Test

Directions: Each of the numbered items or incomplete statements in this section is followed by answers or by completions of the statement. Select the **one** lettered answer or completion that is **best** in each case.

1. Which germ layers are present at the end of week 3 of development (day 21)?

(A) Epiblast only
(B) Epiblast and hypoblast
(C) Ectoderm and endoderm
(D) Ectoderm, mesoderm, and endoderm
(E) Epiblast, mesoderm, and hypoblast

2. Which process establishes the three definitive germ layers?

(A) Neurulation
(B) Gastrulation
(C) Craniocaudal folding
(D) Lateral folding
(E) Angiogenesis

3. The first indication of gastrulation in the embryo is

(A) formation of the primitive streak
(B) formation of the notochord
(C) formation of the neural tube
(D) formation of extraembryonic mesoderm
(E) formation of tertiary chorionic villi

4. Somites may differentiate into all of the following EXCEPT

(A) bone
(B) cartilage
(C) muscle
(D) epidermis of skin
(E) dermis of skin

5. Intermediate mesoderm will give rise to the

(A) neural tube
(B) heart
(C) kidneys and gonads
(D) somites
(E) notochord

6. The developing embryo has a distinct human appearance by the end of

(A) week 4
(B) week 5
(C) week 6
(D) week 7
(E) week 8

7. The lateral mesoderm is divided into two distinct layers by the formation of the

(A) extraembryonic coelom
(B) intraembryonic coelom
(C) cardiogenic region
(D) notochord
(E) yolk sac

8. All of the following statements concerning the notochord are true EXCEPT

(A) it induces overlying ectoderm to form the neural plate
(B) it induces the formation of vertebral bodies
(C) it forms the nucleus pulposus
(D) it forms the neural tube
(E) it extends from the primitive node to the prochordal plate

9. Very often the first indication a woman has that she is pregnant is a missed menstrual period. In which week of embryonic development will a woman experience her first missed menstrual period?

(A) Start of week 3
(B) Start of week 4
(C) Start of week 5
(D) Start of week 8
(E) End of week 8

10. A female newborn was found to have a large midline tumor in the lower sacral area, which was diagnosed as a sacrococcygeal tumor. Which of the following courses of treatment is recommended for this child?

(A) Immediate chemotherapy and radiation treatment
(B) Surgical removal by age 6 months
(C) Surgical removal at age 4–5 years
(D) Surgical removal at age 13–15 years
(E) No treatment because this tumor normally regresses with age

11. A woman has her pregnancy suddenly terminated due to intrauterine fetal death. At autopsy, the fetus shows severe pallor, generalized edema, and hepatosplenomegaly. Which of the following would you suspect?

(A) VATER
(B) β-thalassemia minor
(C) β-thalassemia major
(D) Hydrops fetalis
(E) VACTERL

Answers and Explanations

1–D. During week 3 of development, the process of gastrulation, which establishes the three primary germ layers (ectoderm, intraembryonic mesoderm, and endoderm), occurs. The origin of all tissues and organs of the adult can be traced to one of these germ layers since these tissues and organs "germinate" from these germ layers.

2–B. Gastrulation establishes the three primary germ layers during week 3 of development. Neurulation is the process by which neuroectoderm forms the neural plate, which eventually folds to form the neural tube.

3–A. The formation of the primitive streak on the dorsal surface of the bilaminar embryonic disk is the first indication of gastrulation.

4–D. Approximately 35 pairs of somites form; they are derived from a specific subdivision of intraembryonic mesoderm called paraxial mesoderm. Somites differentiate into the components called sclerotome (cartilage and bone), myotome (muscle), and dermatome (dermis of skin). The epidermis of skin (stratified squamous epithelium) is derived from ectoderm.

5–C. Intermediate mesoderm is a subdivision of intraembryonic mesoderm that forms a longitudinal dorsal ridge, called the urogenital ridge, from which the kidneys and gonads develop.

6–E. The embryo starts the embryonic period as a two-dimensional disk and ends as a three-dimensional cylinder. This dramatic change in geometry is caused by formation of all the major organ systems. As the organ systems gradually develop during the embryonic period, the embryo appears more and more humanlike; it has a distinct human appearance at the end of week 8.

7–B. The lateral mesoderm is a subdivision of intraembryonic mesoderm and initially is a solid plate of mesoderm. The intraembryonic coelom forms in the middle of the lateral mesoderm, thereby dividing it into the intraembryonic somatic mesoderm and intraembryonic visceral mesoderm.

8–D. The notochord, which extends from the primitive node to the prochordal plate, does not develop into any part of the neural tube [or thereby the central nervous system (CNS)]. The relationship of the notochord to the CNS is purely inductive; ectoderm overlying the notochord is induced to form the neural plate. Other roles of the notochord include inducing the formation of vertebral bodies and formation of the nucleus pulposus.

9–A. Assuming a regular 28-day menstrual cycle, a woman will start menses on February 1, for example. On February 14, she will ovulate, and the secondary oocyte is fertilized within 24 hours. So, the zygote undergoes week 1 of development from February 15 to 21. Week 2 of development is from February 22 to 28. On March 1, the woman should enter her next menstrual cycle, but because she is pregnant, she will not menstruate. Therefore, this first missed menstrual period corresponds with the start of week 3 of embryonic development. The embryonic period (week 3 to week 8) is a time of high susceptibility to teratogens.

10–B. The preponderance of sacrococcygeal tumors is found in female newborns. Since these tumors develop from pluripotent cells of primitive streak origin, malignancy is of great concern, and the tumor should be surgically removed by age 6 months. Occasionally, these tumors may recur after surgery, demonstrating malignant properties.

11–D. Hydrops fetalis is the most severe form of α-thalassemia, which is a direct result of the lack or decreased synthesis of the α-globin chain of hemoglobin $\alpha_2\gamma_2$.

5

Cardiovascular System

I. Development of the Heart

A. Formation of the heart tube (Figure 5-1)

1. Lateral plate mesoderm (at the cephalic area of the embryo) will split into a **somatic layer** and **splanchnic layer**, thus forming the **pericardial cavity**. Pre-cardiac mesoderm is preferentially distributed to the splanchnic layer and is now called **heart-forming regions (HFRs).**

2. As lateral folding of the embryo occurs, the HFRs will fuse in the midline to form a continuous sheet of mesoderm.

3. Hypertrophied foregut endoderm secretes **vascular endothelial growth factor (VEGF)** that induces the sheet of **mesoderm** to form discontinuous vascular channels that eventually get remodeled into a single endocardial tube (**endocardium**).

4. Mesoderm around the endocardium forms the **myocardium**, which secretes a layer of extracellular matrix proteins called **cardiac jelly**.

5. Mesoderm migrating into the cardiac region from the coelomic wall near the liver forms the **epicardium**.

B. Primitive heart tube dilatations (Figure 5-2)

1. Five dilatations soon become apparent along the length of the tube: **truncus arteriosus (T), bulbus cordis (B), primitive ventricle (PV), primitive atrium (PA),** and **sinus venosus (SV).**

2. These five embryonic dilatations develop into the adult structures of the heart (Table 5-1).

C. Dextral looping (Figure 5-3)

1. In the primitive heart tube, venous blood flows through the left ventricle *prior to* the right ventricle. This situation must be corrected since in the normal adult heart venous blood flows into the right ventricle.

2. Dextral looping is the key event in this correction such that the location of the **atrioventricular canal** and the **conoventricular canal** become properly aligned.

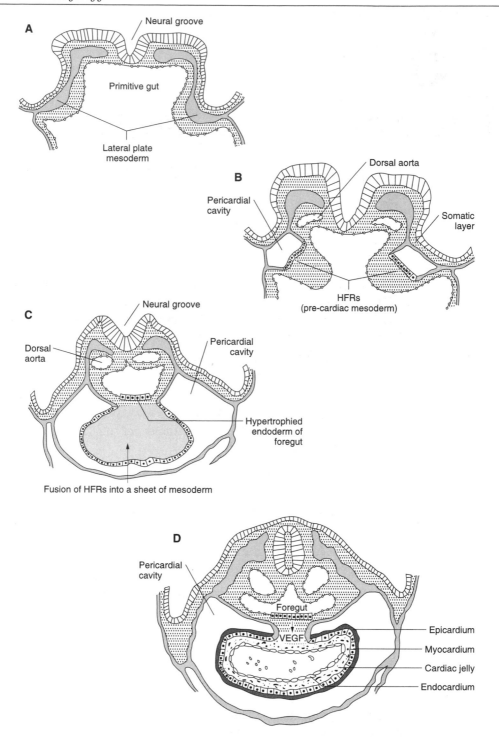

Figure 5-1. A schematic diagram depicting cross sections of an embryo at the level of the developing heart. *(A)* Formation of lateral plate mesoderm. *(B)* Splitting of lateral plate mesoderm. *(C)* Fusion of heart-forming regions (HFRs) in the midline into a sheet of mesoderm. *(D)* Vascular endothelial growth factor (VEGF) induction of single endocardial tube.

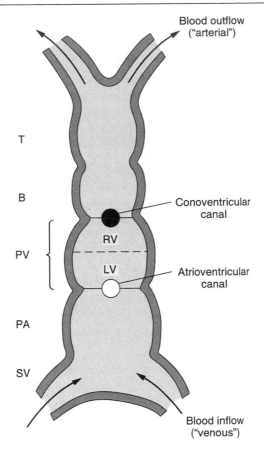

Figure 5-2. A schematic diagram depicting the primitive heart tube and its five dilatations. Note the location of the atrioventricular canal and conoventricular canal. *Arrows* show the direction of blood flow from the "venous" blood inflow at the sinus venosus to the "arterial" blood outflow at the truncus arteriosus. Note that "venous" blood inflow enters the left ventricle (LV) before it enters the right ventricle (RV). *B* = bulbus cordis; *PA* = primitive atrium; *PV* = primitive ventricle; *SV* = sinus venosus; *T* = truncus arteriosus.

    a. Early looping seems to be inherently programmed within the myocardial cells.

    b. Convergence begins to bring the atrioventricular canal and the conoventricular canal into proper alignment.

    c. Wedging causes the conoventricular canal to nestle between the tricuspid and mitral valves and occurs concurrently with the formation of the aorticopulmonary (AP) septum.

    d. Repositioning causes the atrioventricular canal to straddle both the right and left ventricles.

D. Formation of the aorticopulmonary (AP) septum (Figure 5-4)

    1. Neural crest cells migrate from the hindbrain region through pharyngeal arches 3, 4, and 6 and invade both the **truncal ridges** and **bulbar ridges**.

    2. The truncal and bulbar ridges grow and twist around each other in a spiral fashion and eventually fuse to form the AP septum.

Table 5-1. Correspondence of Embryonic Dilatations and Adult Heart Structures

Embryonic Dilatation	Adult Structure
Truncus arteriosus	Aorta Pulmonary trunk
Bulbus cordis	Smooth part of right ventricle (conus arteriosus) Smooth part of left ventricle (aortic vestibule)
Primitive ventricle	Trabeculated part of right ventricle Trabeculated part of left ventricle
Primitive atrium	Trabeculated part of right atrium Trabeculated part of left atrium
Sinus venosus	Smooth part of right atrium (sinus venarum)*† Coronary sinus Oblique vein of left atrium

* The smooth part of the left atrium is formed by incorporation of parts of the **pulmonary veins** into its wall.
† The junction of the trabeculated and smooth parts of the right atrium is called **crista terminalis.**

3. The AP septum divides the truncus arteriosus and bulbus cordis into the aorta and pulmonary trunk.

E. Formation of the atrial septum (Figure 5-5)

1. The crescent-shaped **septum primum** forms in the roof of the primitive atrium and grows toward the atrioventricular (AV) cushions in the AV canal.

2. The **foramen primum** forms between the free edge of the septum primum and the AV cushions; it is closed when the septum primum fuses with the AV cushions.

3. The **foramen secundum** forms in the center of the septum primum.

4. The crescent-shaped **septum secundum** forms to the right of the septum primum.

5. The **foramen ovale** is the opening between the upper and lower limbs of the septum secundum.

   a. During embryonic life, blood is shunted from the right atrium to the left atrium via the foramen ovale.

   b. Immediately after birth, functional closure of the foramen ovale is facilitated both by a decrease in right atrial pressure from occlusion of placental circulation and by an increase in left atrial pressure due to increased pulmonary venous return.

6. Later in life, the septum primum and septum secundum anatomically fuse to complete the formation of the atrial septum.

F. Formation of the atrioventricular (AV) septum (Figure 5-6)

1. The **dorsal AV cushion** and **ventral AV cushion** approach each other and fuse to form the AV septum.

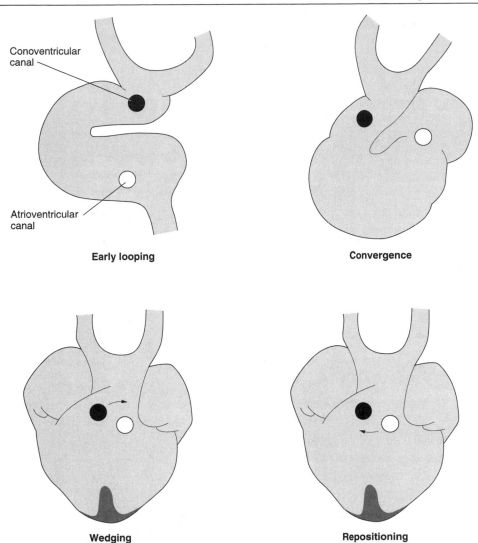

Figure 5-3. A schematic diagram depicting dextral looping. Note the change in the location of both the atrioventricular canal and the conoventricular canal.

  2. The AV septum partitions the AV canal into the right AV canal and left AV canal.

G. Formation of the interventricular (IV) septum (Figure 5-7)

  1. The **muscular IV septum** develops in the midline on the floor of the primitive ventricle and grows toward the fused AV cushions.

  2. The **IV foramen** is located between the free edge of the muscular IV septum and the fused AV cushions.

  3. This foramen is closed by the **membranous IV septum,** which forms by the proliferation and fusion of tissue from three sources: the **right bulbar ridge, left bulbar ridge,** and **AV cushions.**

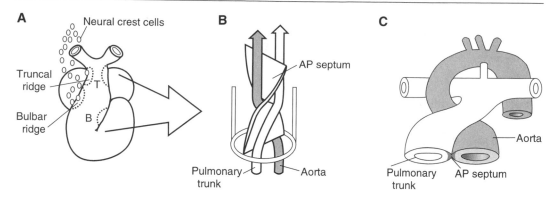

Figure 5-4. Formation of the AP septum. *(A)* Partitioning of the truncus arteriosus and bulbus cordis, involving neural crest cell migration. *(B)* The aorticopulmonary septum develops in a spiral fashion. *(C)* The spiral aorticopulmonary septum accounts for the adult gross anatomic relationship between the aorta *(shaded)* and pulmonary trunk *(unshaded)*. *AP* = aorticopulmonary; *B* = bulbus cordis; *T* = truncus arteriosus.

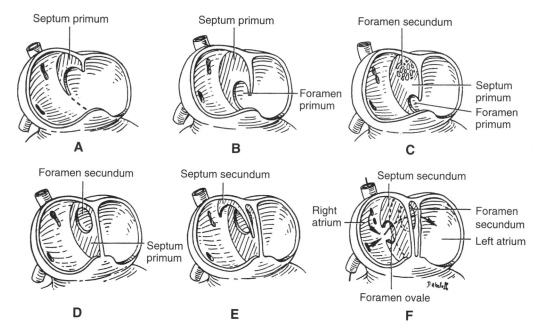

Figure 5-5. Formation of the atrial septum. The *arrows* in *F* indicate the direction of blood flow across the fully developed septum, from the right atrium to the left atrium. (Modified with permission from Johnson KE: *NMS Human Developmental Anatomy.* Baltimore, Williams & Wilkins, 1988, p. 149.)

H. The conduction system of the heart

1. At week 5, cardiac myocytes in the sinus venosus region of the primitive heart tube begin to undergo spontaneous electrical depolarizations at a rate *faster* than cardiac myocytes in other regions. As dextral looping occurs, the sinus venosus becomes incorporated into the right atrium and these fast depolarizing cardiac myocytes become the **sinoatrial (SA) node** and the **atrioventricular (AV) node.** In the adult, the cardiac myocytes of the SA and AV nodes remain committed to fast electrical depolarizations instead of developing contractile properties.

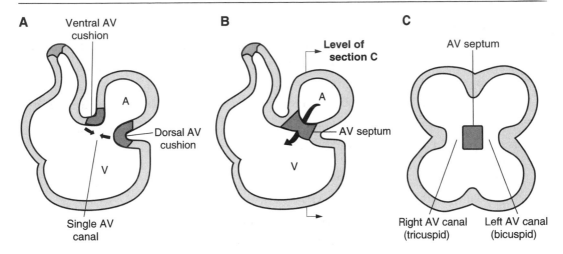

Figure 5-6. Formation of the AV septum. *(A–C)* Partitioning of the atrioventricular canal. A = atrium; AV = atrioventricular; V = ventricle.

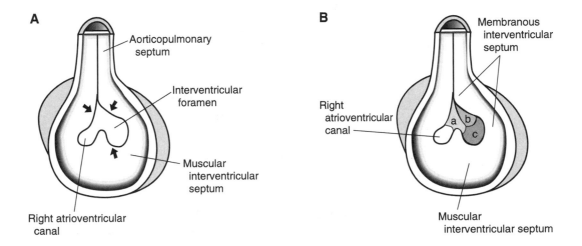

Figure 5-7. Formation of the interventricular (IV) septum. *(A and B)* Partitioning of the primitive ventricle. *Shaded portion (a, b, c)* in *B* indicates the three sources of the membranous interventricular septum. *a* = right bulbar ridge; *b* = left bulbar ridge; *c* = atrioventricular (AV) cushions.

2. As the atria and ventricles become electrically isolated by the formation of the fibrous skeleton of the heart, the **AV node** provides the *only* pathway for depolarizations to flow from the atria to ventricles.

3. The **AV bundle** or **bundle of His** develops from a ring-like cluster of cells found at the AV junction that specifically expresses the homeobox gene, ***msx-2.***

4. The **intramural network of Purkinje myocytes** has a distinct embryological origin (versus the Bundle of His) in that Purkinje myocytes develop from already contractile cardiac myocytes within the myocardium and can therefore be considered as **modified cardiac myocytes.**

I. Coronary arteries

1. Progenitor stem cells from the liver migrate into the primitive heart tube and take residence beneath the epicaridium.

2. These progenitor stem cells form vascular channels that grow towards the truncus arteriosus (future aorta) and form a **peritruncal capillary ring**.

3. Only two of these capillaries survive and these become the proximal portions of the right and left coronary arteries.

J. Clinical considerations

1. Aorticopulmonary (AP) septal defects (Figure 5-8)

a. Persistent truncus arteriosus (PTA)

– is caused by abnormal neural crest cell migration such that there is only *partial* development of the AP septum.
– results in a condition in which one large vessel leaves the heart and receives blood from both the right and left ventricles.
– is usually accompanied by a membranous VSD.
– is associated clinically with marked cyanosis.

b. D-Transposition of the great arteries (complete)

– is caused by abnormal neural crest cell migration such that there is *non-spiral* development of the AP septum.
– results in a condition in which the aorta arises abnormally from the *right* ventricle, and the pulmonary trunk arises abnormally from the *left* ventricle; hence the systemic and pulmonary circulations are *completely* separated from each other.
– is incompatible with life unless an accompanying shunt such as a VSD, patent foramen ovale, or patent ductus arteriosus exists.
– is associated clinically with marked cyanosis.

c. L-Transposition of the great vessels (corrected)

– The aorta and pulmonary trunk are transposed and the ventricles are "inverted" such that the anatomical right ventricle lies on the left side and the anatomical left ventricle lies on the right side.
– These two major deviations offset one another such that blood flow pattern is normal.

d. Double outlet right ventricle (DORV or incomplete transposition)

– The aorta and pulmonary trunk both arise primarily from the right ventricle.
– is usually associated with a VSD that provides the only outlet for blood in the left ventricle.

e. Tetralogy of Fallot

– is caused by an abnormal neural crest cell migration such that there is *skewed* development of the AP septum.
– results in a condition in which the pulmonary trunk obtains a small diameter while the aorta obtains a large diameter.
– is associated clinically with marked cyanosis.

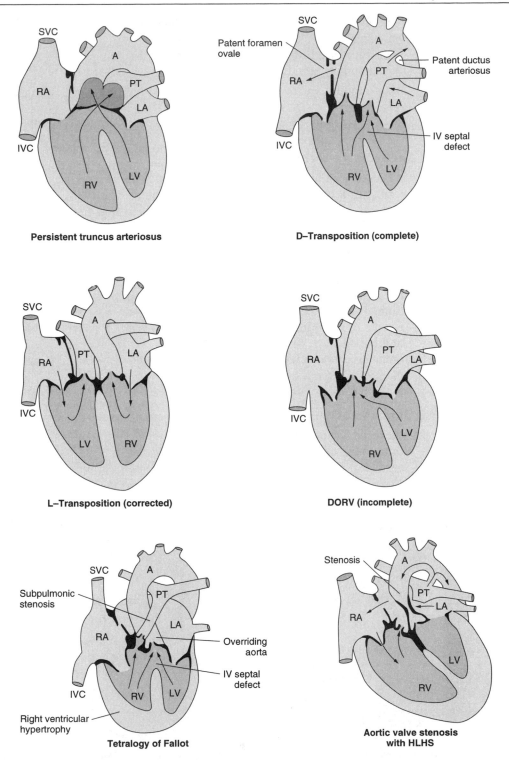

Figure 5-8. Aorticopulmonary (AP) septal defects. *Arrows* indicate direction of blood flow. *A* = aorta; *DORV* = double outlet right ventricle; *HLHS* = hypoplastic left heart syndrome; *IV* = interventricular; *IVC* = inferior vena cava; *LA* = left atrium; *LV* = left ventricle; *PT* = pulmonary trunk; *RA* = right atrium; *RV* = right ventricle; *SVC* = superior vena cava.

– The clinical consequences depend primarily on the severity of the pulmonary stenosis.

– is characterized by four classic malformations:

(1) Pulmonary stenosis

(2) Overriding aorta

(3) VSD

(4) Right ventricular hypertrophy

f. Aortic valve stenosis

– is caused by the fusion of the cusps of the semilunar valve.

– results in a condition in which left ventricular blood outflow may be severely restricted, leading to **hypoplastic left heart syndrome (HLHS)**.

2. Atrial septal defects (ASDs; Figure 5-9)

a. Foramen secundum defect

– is caused by excessive resorption of septum primum, septum secundum, or both.

– results in a condition in which there is an opening between the right and left atria.

– Some defects can be tolerated for a long time, with clinical symptoms manifesting as late as age 30.

– is the most common clinically significant ASD.

b. Common atrium (cor triloculare biventriculare)

– is caused by the complete failure of septum primum and septum secundum to develop.

– results in a condition in which there is formation of only one atrium.

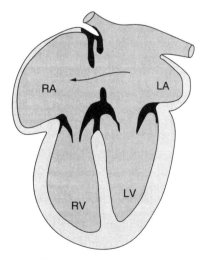

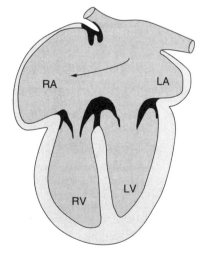

Foramen secundum defect

Common atrium
(cor triloculare biventriculare)

Figure 5-9. Atrial septal defects (ASDs). *Arrows* indicate direction of blood flow. *LA* = left atrium; *LV* = left ventricle; *RA* = right atrium; *RV* = right ventricle.

c. Probe patency of the foramen ovale

- is caused by incomplete anatomic fusion of septum primum and septum secundum.
- is present in approximately 25% of the population.
- is usually of no clinical importance.

d. Premature closure of foramen ovale

- is closure of foramen ovale during prenatal life.
- results in hypertrophy of the right side of the heart and underdevelopment of the left side of the heart.

3. Atrioventricular (AV) septal defects (Figure 5-10)

a. Persistent common AV canal

- is caused by *failure of fusion* of the dorsal and ventral AV cushions.
- results in a condition in which the common AV canal is never partitioned into the right and left AV canals, resulting in a large hole in the center of the heart.
- Tricuspid and bicuspid valves are represented by one valve common to both sides of the heart.
- Two common hemodynamic abnormalities are found:

(1) L→R shunt of blood from the left atrium to the right atrium causing an enlarged right atrium and right ventricle

(2) Mitral valve regurgitation causing an enlarged left atrium and left ventricle

b. Foramen primum defect

- is caused by a failure of the AV septum to fuse with septum primum.
- results in a condition in which the foramen primum is never closed.
- is generally accompanied by an abnormal mitral valve.

c. Ebstein's anomaly

- is caused by the failure of the posterior and septal leaflets of the tricuspid valve to attach normally to the annulus fibrosus but are instead displaced inferiorly into the right ventricle.
- results in a condition in which the right ventricle is divided into a large, upper, "atrialized" portion and a small, lower, functional portion.
- Due to the small, functional portion of the right ventricle, there is a reduced amount of blood available to the pulmonary trunk.
- is usually associated with an ASD.

d. Univentricular heart

- is caused by an extremly skewed development of the AV septum to the right.
- results in a condition in which there is one ventricle that receives both the tricuspid and mitral valves.
- is usually associated with a VSD.

e. Tricuspid atresia (hypoplastic right heart)

- is caused by an insufficient amount of AV cushion tissue available for the formation of the tricuspid valve.

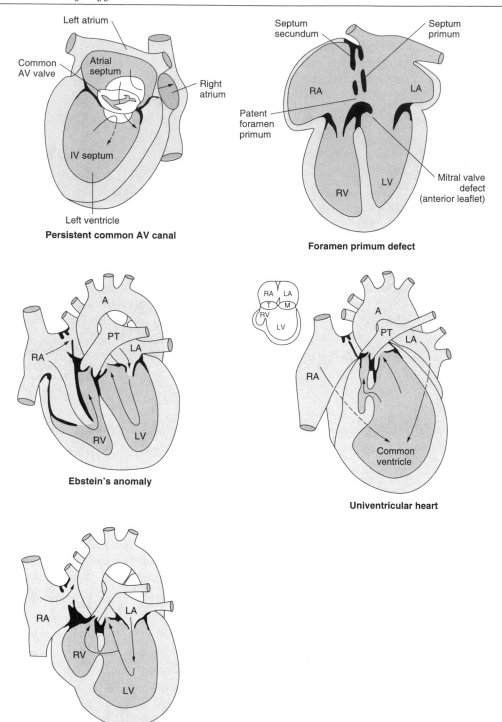

Figure 5-10. Atrioventricular (AV) septal defects. *Arrows* indicate direction of blood flow. *A* = aorta; *LA* = left atrium; *LV* = left ventricle; *PT* = pulmonary trunk; *RA* = right atrium; *RV* = right ventricle.

– results in a condition in which there is complete agenesis of the tricuspid valve so that no communication between the right atrium and right ventricle exists.

– is associated clinically with marked cyanosis.

– is always accompanied by the following:

(1) Patent foramen ovale

(2) IV septum defect

(3) Overdeveloped left ventricle

(4) Underdeveloped right ventricle

4. Interventricular (IV) septal defects (VSDs)

a. Membranous VSD (Figure 5-11)

– is caused by faulty fusion of the right bulbar ridge, left bulbar ridge, and AV cushions.

– results in a condition in which an opening between the right and left ventricles allows free flow of blood.

– A large VSD is initially associated with a L→R shunting of blood, increased pulmonary blood flow, and pulmonary hypertension.

– One of the secondary effects of a large VSD and its associated pulmonary hypertension is proliferation of the tunica intima and tunica media of pulmonary muscular arteries and arterioles, resulting in a narrowing of their lumen. Ultimately, pulmonary resistance may become higher than systemic resistance and cause R→L shunting of blood and cyanosis. At this stage, the characteristic of the patient has been termed the "**Eisenmenger complex**."

– is the most common type of VSD.

b. Muscular VSD

– is caused by single or multiple perforations in the muscular IV septum.

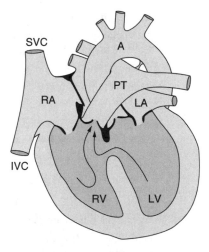

Membranous VSD

Figure 5-11. Interventricular (IV) septal defects showing a membranous ventricular septal defect (VSD). *Arrows* indicate direction of blood flow. *A* = aorta; *IVC* = inferior vena cava; *LA* = left atrium; *LV* = left ventricle; *PT* = pulmonary trunk; *RA* = right atrium; *RV* = right ventricle; *SVC* = superior vena cava.

c. **Common ventricle (cor triloculare biatriatum)**

  – is caused by failure of the membranous and muscular IV septa to form.

5. **Abnormal positions of the heart**

  a. **Isolated dextrocardia**

  – The heart is abnormally positioned on the right side of the thorax.
  – is usually associated with other severe cardiac anomalies.

  b. **Dextrocardia with situs inversus**

  – is dextrocardia with inversion of the viscera (for example, liver on the left side).
  – is not usually associated with other severe cardiac anomalies.

II. Development of the Arterial System (Table 5-2)

A. **General pattern**

  – develops mainly from 6 pairs of arteries (called **aortic arches**) that course through the pharyngeal arches and the **right** and **left dorsal aortae**.
  – The aortic arch arteries undergo remodeling.
  – The right and left dorsal aortae fuse to form the **dorsal aorta**, which then sprouts **posterolateral arteries, lateral arteries,** and **ventral arteries (vitelline** and **umbilical).**

Table 5-2. Correspondence of Embryonic and Adult Arteries

Embryonic	Adult
Aortic Arch Arteries	
1	Maxillary artery (portion of)
2	Stapedial artery (portion of)
3	Right and left common carotid arteries (portion of)
	Right and left internal carotid arteries
4	Right subclavian artery (portion of)
	Arch of the aorta (portion of)
5	Regresses in the human
6*	Right and left pulmonary arteries (portion of)
	Ductus arteriosus
Dorsal Aorta	
Posterolateral arteries	Arteries to the upper and lower extremities
	Intercostal, lumbar, and lateral sacral arteries
Lateral arteries	Renal, suprarenal, and gonadal arteries
Ventral arteries	
Vitelline	Celiac, superior mesenteric, and inferior mesenteric arteries
Umbilical	Internal iliac (portion of) and superior vesical arteries
	Medial umbilical ligaments

* Early in development, the recurrent laryngeal nerves hook around aortic arch 6. On the right side, the distal part of aortic arch 6 regresses, and the right recurrent laryngeal nerve moves up to hook around the right subclavian artery. On the left side, aortic arch 6 persists as the ductus arteriosus (or ligamentum arteriosus in the adult); the left recurrent laryngeal nerve remains hooked around the ductus arteriosus.

B. Clinical considerations

– Most anomalies of the great arteries occur as a result of persistence of parts of the aortic arch system that normally regress and regression of parts that normally persist

1. Abnormal origin of the right subclavian artery

– occurs when right aortic arch 4 and the right dorsal aorta cranial to the seventh intersegmental artery abnormally regress.
– As development continues, the right subclavian artery will come to lie on the *left* side just inferior to the left subclavian artery.
– The artery must cross the midline posterior to the trachea and esophagus to supply the right arm.
– may constrict the trachea or esophagus; generally is not clinically significant.

2. Double aortic arch

– occurs when an abnormal right aortic arch develops in addition to a left aortic arch due to persistence of the distal portion of the right dorsal aorta.
– forms a vascular ring around the trachea and esophagus, which causes difficulties in breathing and swallowing.

3. Right aortic arch

– occurs when the entire right dorsal aorta abnormally persists and part of the left dorsal aorta regresses.
– The right aortic arch may pass anterior or posterior (retroesophageal right arch) to the esophagus and trachea. A retroesophageal right arch may cause difficulties in swallowing or breathing.

4. Postductal coarctation of the aorta (Figure 5-12A)

– occurs when the aorta is abnormally constricted; cause is unclear.
– is found distal to the origin of the left subclavian artery and inferior to the ductus arteriosus.

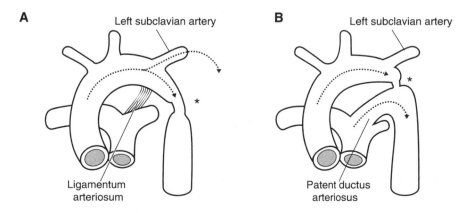

Figure 5-12. Coarctation of the aorta. *(A)* Postductal: Blood reaches lower part of the body via collateral circulation through the left subclavian, intercostal, and internal thoracic arteries. *(B)* Preductal: Blood reaches lower part of the body through a patent ductus arteriosus. *Asterisk* (*) indicates point of constriction. *Dotted arrows* indicate direction of blood flow.

– is clinically associated with increased blood pressure in the upper extremities, lack of pulse in femoral artery, and high risk of both cerebral hemorrhage and bacterial endocarditis.

– is commonly associated with Turner syndrome.

– Less commonly, a coarctation may occur superior to the ductus arteriosus (**preductal**; see Figure 5-12*B*).

5. Patent ductus arteriosus

– occurs when the ductus arteriosus, a connection between the pulmonary artery and aorta, fails to close; normally it functionally closes within a few hours after birth via smooth muscle contraction to ultimately form the **ligamentum arteriosum**.

– causes a shunting of oxygen-rich blood from the aorta back into the pulmonary circulation.

– can be treated with prostaglandin synthesis inhibitors (such as indomethacin), which promote closure.

– is very common in premature infants and maternal rubella infection.

III. Development of the Venous System (Table 5-3)

A. General pattern

– develops mainly from three pairs of veins: the **vitelline veins, umbilical veins,** and **cardinal veins** that empty blood into the sinus venosus.

– These veins undergo remodeling due to a L→R shunting of venous blood to the right atrium.

Table 5-3. Correspondence of Embryonic and Adult Veins

Embryonic	Adult
Vitelline Veins	
Right and left	Portion of the IVC
	Hepatic veins and sinusoids
	Ductus venosus
	Portal vein
	Inferior mesenteric vein
	Superior mesenteric vein
	Splenic vein
Umbilical Veins	
Right	Degenerates early in fetal life
Left	Ligamentum teres
Cardinal Veins	
Anterior	SVC, internal jugular veins
Posterior	Portion of IVC, common iliac veins
Subcardinal	Portion of IVC, renal veins, gonadal veins
Supracardinal	Portion of IVC, intercostal veins, hemiazygos vein, azygos vein

IVC = inferior vena cava (note that the IVC is derived embryologically from four different sources); *SVC* = superior vena cava.

B. Clinical considerations

– Most anomalies of the venous system occur as a result of persistence of the veins on the left side of the body that normally regress during the left-to-right shunting of blood.

1. Double inferior vena cava

– occurs when the left supracardinal vein persists, thereby forming an additional inferior vena cava below the level of the kidneys.

2. Left superior vena cava

– occurs when the left anterior cardinal vein persists, forming a superior vena cava on the left side; the right anterior cardinal vein abnormally regresses.

3. Double superior vena cava

– occurs when the left anterior cardinal vein persists, forming a superior vena cava on the left side; the right anterior cardinal vein also forms a superior vena cava on the right side.

4. Absence of the hepatic portion of the inferior vena cava

– occurs when the right vitelline vein fails to form a segment of the inferior vena cava.
– Consequently, blood from the lower part of the body reaches the right atrium via the azygos vein, hemiazygos vein, and superior vena cava.

Review Test

Directions: Each of the numbered items or incomplete statements in this section is followed by answers or by completions of the statement. Select the **one** lettered answer or completion that is **best** in each case.

1. The most common interventricular septal defect (VSD) seen clinically is

(A) persistent truncus arteriosus
(B) membranous VSD
(C) common ventricle
(D) foramen secundum defect
(E) premature closure of foramen ovale

2. Which of the following clinical signs would be most obvious on examination of a patient with either tetralogy of Fallot or transposition of the great vessels?

(A) Sweaty palms
(B) Lack of femoral artery pulse
(C) Pulmonary hypertension
(D) Cyanosis
(E) Diffuse red rash

3. Which of the following congenital cardiovascular malformations is most commonly associated with maternal rubella infection?

(A) Isolated dextrocardia
(B) Patent ductus arteriosus
(C) Persistent truncus arteriosus
(D) Coarctation of the aorta
(E) Double aortic arch

4. The most common atrial septal defect (ASD) seen clinically is

(A) common atrium
(B) foramen secundum defect
(C) premature closure of the foramen ovale
(D) persistent truncus arteriosus
(E) probe patency of the foramen ovale

5. The ventral surface of the adult heart as seen on gross examination or radiography is comprised primarily of the

(A) left atrium
(B) left ventricle
(C) inferior vena cava
(D) bulbus cordis
(E) right ventricle

6. The left recurrent laryngeal nerve recurs around the

(A) left primary bronchus
(B) left subclavian artery
(C) left subclavian vein
(D) ductus arteriosus
(E) left common carotid artery

7. Which of the three primary germ layers forms the histologically definitive endocardium of the adult heart?

(A) Ectoderm
(B) Endoderm
(C) Mesoderm
(D) Epiblast
(E) Hypoblast

8. Which of the following is responsible for the proper alignment of the atrioventricular canal and the conoventricular canal?

(A) Lateral folding of the embryo
(B) Craniocaudal folding of the embryo
(C) Programmed cell migration
(D) Formation of the aorticopulmonary (AP) septum
(E) Dextral looping

9. All of the following cardiac malformations are clinically associated with cyanosis EXCEPT

(A) transposition of the great arteries
(B) tetralogy of Fallot
(C) tricuspid atresia
(D) membranous ventricular septal defect (VSD)
(E) persistent truncus arteriosus

58

10. Tricuspid atresia is characterized by the obliteration of the right atrioventricular canal and by the absence of the tricuspid valve. All of the following defects are associated with tricuspid atresia EXCEPT

(A) patent foramen ovale
(B) overriding aorta
(C) interventricular septal defect
(D) overdeveloped left ventricle
(E) underdeveloped right ventricle

11. The hepatic sinusoids that can be observed histologically in an adult liver are derived from the

(A) umbilical veins
(B) anterior cardinal veins
(C) posterior cardinal veins
(D) vitelline veins
(E) subcardinal veins

12. Which of the following arterial malformations is very common in premature infants?

(A) Patent ductus arteriosus
(B) Coarctation of the aorta
(C) Right aortic arch
(D) Double aortic arch
(E) Abnormal origin of the right subclavian artery

13. A physician monitoring a newborn infant's heart sounds using a stethoscope hears the characteristic murmur of a patent ductus arteriosus. How soon after birth should this murmur normally disappear?

(A) 1–2 months
(B) 1–2 weeks
(C) 1–2 days
(D) 1–2 hours
(E) Immediately

14. How soon after birth does the foramen ovale close?

(A) 1–2 months
(B) 1–2 weeks
(C) 1–2 days
(D) 1–2 hours
(E) Immediately

15. A 9-year-old boy presents with complaints of numbness and tingling in both feet. Examination reveals no pulse in the femoral artery, increased blood pressure in the arteries of the upper extremity, and enlarged intercostal veins. Which of the following abnormalities would be suspected?

(A) Double aortic arch
(B) Tetralogy of Fallot
(C) Postductal coarctation of the aorta
(D) Right aortic arch
(E) Abnormal origin of the right subclavian artery

16. The inferior vena cava is formed from all of the following embryonic veins EXCEPT

(A) vitelline veins
(B) umbilical veins
(C) posterior cardinal veins
(D) subcardinal veins
(E) supracardinal veins

Directions: Each group of items in this section consists of lettered options followed by a set of numbered items. For each item, select the **one** lettered option that is most closely associated with it. Each lettered option may be selected once, more than once, or not at all.

Questions 17–27

Match each definitive adult structure below with the most appropriate embryonic heart dilatation.

(A) Truncus arteriosus
(B) Bulbus cordis
(C) Primitive ventricle
(D) Primitive atrium
(E) Sinus venosus
(F) None of the above

17. Coronary sinus

18. Conus arteriosus

19. Proximal part of aorta

20. Aortic vestibule

21. Sinus venarum

22. Trabeculated part of right ventricle

23. Trabeculated part of right atrium

24. Inferior vena cava

25. Proximal part of pulmonary artery

26. Smooth part of left atrium

27. Superior vena cava

Questions 28–37

Match each cardiac malformation below with the most appropriate septum.

(A) Aorticopulmonary septum
(B) Atrial septum
(C) Atrioventricular septum
(D) Interventricular septum

28. Common ventricle

29. Tricuspid atresia

30. Muscular ventricular septal defect (VSD)

31. Foramen primum defect

32. Tetralogy of Fallot

33. Foramen secundum defect

34. Probe patency of the foramen ovale

35. Membranous ventricular septal defect (VSD)

36. Aortic valve stenosis

37. Persistent truncus arteriosus

Questions 38–46

Match each of the following causes with the most appropriate cardiac malformation.

(A) Persistent truncus arteriosus (PTA)
(B) Univentricular heart
(C) Transposition of the great arteries
(D) Aortic valve stenosis
(E) Foramen secundum defect
(F) Persistent common atrioventricular (AV) canal
(G) Tricuspid atresia
(H) Membranous ventricular septal defect (VSD)
(I) Tetralogy of Fallot

38. Skewed development of the aorticopulmonary (AP) septum

39. Failure of fusion of atrioventricular (AV) cushions

40. Insufficient amount of atrioventricular (AV) cushion tissue

41. Partial development of aorticopulmonary (AP) septum

42. Skewed development of the atrioventricular (AV) septum

43. Faulty fusion of the right and left bulbar ridges and atrioventricular (AV) cushion

44. Non-spiral development of aorticopulmonary (AP) septum

45. Excessive resorption of septum primum or septum secundum

46. Fusion of the semilunar valve cusps in the aorta

Questions 47–53

Match each definitive adult artery below with the most appropriate arterial branch of the dorsal aorta.

(A) Posterolateral arteries
(B) Lateral arteries
(C) Ventral arteries

47. Renal arteries

48. Intercostal arteries

49. Celiac artery

50. Superior mesenteric artery

51. Internal iliac arteries

52. Arteries to upper extremity

53. Gonadal arteries

Questions 54–60

Match each definitive adult artery below with the most appropriate aortic arch.

(A) Aortic arch 1
(B) Aortic arch 2
(C) Aortic arch 3
(D) Aortic arch 4
(E) Aortic arch 5
(F) Aortic arch 6

54. Internal carotid artery

55. Arch of the aorta

56. Stapedial artery

57. Left pulmonary artery

58. Right subclavian artery

59. Common carotid artery

60. Right pulmonary artery

Questions 61–68

Match each definitive adult vein below with the most appropriate embryonic vein.

(A) Vitelline veins
(B) Umbilical veins
(C) Anterior cardinal veins
(D) Posterior cardinal veins
(E) Subcardinal veins
(F) Supracardinal veins

61. Portal vein

62. Internal jugular veins

63. Azygos vein

64. Renal veins

65. Superior vena cava

66. Hemiazygos vein

67. Superior mesenteric vein

68. Common iliac veins

Answers and Explanations

1–B. The most common of all cardiac congenital malformations seen clinically are membranous ventricular septal defects (VSDs). The membranous interventricular septum forms by the proliferation and fusion of tissue from three different sources: the right and left bulbar ridges and the atrioventricular (AV) cushions. Because of this complex formation, the probability of defects is very high.

2–D. Marked cyanosis is a distinct clinical sign in both tetralogy of Fallot and transposition of the great vessels. Any congenital cardiac malformation that allows right-to-left shunting of blood is sometimes called cyanotic heart disease. Right-to-left shunting allows poorly oxygenated blood from the right side of the heart to mix with highly oxygenated blood on the left side of the heart. This causes decreased oxygen tension to peripheral tissues, leading to a characteristic blue tinge (cyanosis) and bulbous thickening of the fingers and toes (clubbing).

3–B. Patent ductus arteriosus (PDA) is the most common congenital cardiac malformation associated with rubella infection of the mother. It is unclear how the rubella virus acts to cause PDA.

4–B. The most common atrial septal defect (ASD) is foramen secundum defect, which is caused by excessive resorption of the septum primum or the septum secundum. This results in an opening between the atria (patent foramen ovale). Some of these defects may remain undiagnosed and may be tolerated for a long time (up to age 30 before the person presents clinically).

5–E. During embryological formation of the heart, the arterial and venous ends of the heart tube are fixed in place. As further growth continues, the heart tube folds to the right. This greatly contributes to the ventral surface of the adult heart being comprised primarily of the right ventricle. The definitive anatomic orientation of the adult heart within the thorax is not at all similar to the strong image we have in our minds of the classic Valentine's Day heart.

6–D. The left recurrent laryngeal nerve recurs around the ductus arteriosus (ligamentum arteriosus in the adult). Early in embryological development, both the right and left recurrent laryngeal nerves hook (recur) around aortic arch 6. The left aortic arch 6 persists as the ductus arteriosus.

7–C. The entire cardiovascular system is of mesodermal origin.

8–E. Dextral looping aligns these two canals through early looping, convergence, wedging, and repositioning. This is especially important in correcting the unusual blood flow pattern in the primitive heart tube where venous blood flows into the left ventricle prior to the right ventricle.

9–D. A membranous ventricular septal defect (VSD) causes a left-to-right shunting of blood, so it will not be generally associated with cyanosis. Because the pressure in the left ventricle is high, blood flows from the left ventricle through the interventricular defect into the right ventricle. Left-to-right shunting leads to three unfavorable consequences: The left ventricle must do more work to deliver the same amount of oxygenated blood to the peripheral tissues, blood flow to the lungs is increased, and blood pressure in the pulmonary circulation is increased (pulmonary hypertension). A person with left-to-right shunting complains of excessive fatigue on exertion. Cyanosis is generally associated with right-to-left shunting.

10–B. Overriding aorta is one of the cardiac defects associated with tetralogy of Fallot. The remaining are associated with tricuspid atresia.

11–D. Because of the location of the vitelline veins and the tremendous growth of the developing liver (hepatic diverticulum), the vitelline veins are surrounded by the liver and give rise to the hepatic sinusoids.

12–A. Patent ductus arteriosus (PDA) is very common in premature infants. Infants with birth weight less than 1750 grams typically have a PDA during the first 24 hours postnatally. PDA is more common in female infants than in male infants.

13–D. The ductus arteriosus functionally closes within a few hours (1–2) after birth via smooth muscle contraction of the tunica media. Before birth, the patency of the ductus arteriosus is controlled by the low oxygen content of the blood flowing through it, which in turn stimulates production of prostaglandins, which cause smooth muscle to relax. After birth, the high oxygen content of the blood due to lung ventilation inhibits production of prostaglandins, causing smooth muscle contraction. Premature infants can be treated with prostaglandin synthesis inhibitors (such as indomethacin) to promote closure of the ductus arteriosus.

14–E. The foramen ovale functionally closes almost immediately after birth as pressure in the right atrium decreases and pressure in the left atrium increases, thereby pushing the septum primum against the septum secundum. Anatomic fusion occurs much later in life; over 25% of the population have probe patency of the foramen ovale, in which anatomic fusion does not occur.

15–C. No pulse in the femoral artery, increased blood pressure in the arteries of the upper extremity, enlarged intercostal veins, and numbness and tingling in both feet are clinical symptoms indicative of postductal coarctation of the aorta. Because of the constriction of the aorta, the blood supply to the lower extremity is compromised.

16–B. The definitive adult inferior vena cava is segmentally constructed from four different sources, but the umbilical veins do not contribute to its formation. The right umbilical vein completely regresses, and the left umbilical vein forms a remnant in the adult known as the ligamentum teres.

17–E. The coronary sinus is derived from the sinus venosus.

18–B. The smooth part of the right ventricle, known as the conus arteriosus, is derived from the bulbus cordis.

19–A. The proximal part of the aorta is derived from the truncus arteriosus.

20–B. The smooth part of the left ventricle, known as the aortic vestibule, is derived from the bulbus cordis.

21–E. The smooth part of the right atrium, known as the sinus venarum, is derived from the sinus venosus.

22–C. The trabeculated part of the right ventricle is derived from the primitive ventricle.

23–D. The trabeculated part of the right atrium is derived from the primitive atrium.

24–F. The inferior vena cava is not derived from any of the five primitive heart dilatations. It is segmentally constructed from four different sources: the right vitelline vein, the right subcardinal vein, the right supracardinal vein, and the right and left posterior cardinal veins.

25–A. The proximal part of the pulmonary artery is derived from the truncus arteriosus.

26–F. The smooth part of the left atrium is formed by the incorporation of the four pulmonary veins into its wall.

27–F. The superior vena cava is formed from the right anterior cardinal vein.

28–D. Common ventricle is caused by failure of the membranous and muscular interventricular septum to form.

29–C. Tricuspid atresia involves the atrioventricular septum.

30–D. Muscular ventricular septal defect (VSD) is caused by perforations in the muscular interventricular septum.

31–C. Foramen primum defect involves the atrioventricular septum; it occurs when the atrioventricular (AV) cushions fuse only partially.

32–A. Tetralogy of Fallot involves the aorticopulmonary septum.

33–B. Foramen secundum defect involves the atrial septum.

34–B. Probe patency of the foramen ovale is caused by incomplete anatomic fusion of the septum primum and septum secundum in the atrial septum.

35–D. Membranous ventricular septal defect (VSD) is caused by failure of the membranous interventricular septum to develop.

36–A. Aortic valve stenosis involves the aorticopulmonary septum.

37–A. Persistent truncus arteriosus involves incomplete development of the aorticopulmonary septum.

38–I. A skewed aorticopulmonary (AP) septum will cause tetralogy of Fallot.

39–F. A complete failure of the atrioventricular (AV) cushions to fuse will cause persistent common AV canal.

40–G. Insufficient amount of atrioventricular (AV) cushion material will cause tricuspid atresia.

41–A. Partial development of the aorticopulmonary (AP) septum will cause persistent truncus arteriosus.

42–B. Skewed development of the atrioventricular (AV) septum will cause univentricular heart.

43–H. Faulty fusion of the right and left bulbar ridges and atrioventricular (AV) cushions will cause membranous ventricular septal defect (VSD).

44–C. Non-spiral development of the aorticopulmonary (AP) septum will cause transposition of the great vessels.

45–E. Excessive resorption of the septum primum or the septum secundum will cause foramen secundum defect.

46–D. Fusion of the semilunar valve cusps in the aorta will cause aortic valve stenosis.

47–B. The renal arteries are derived from lateral branches of the dorsal aorta.

48–A. The intercostal arteries are derived from posterolateral branches of the dorsal aorta.

49–C. The celiac artery is derived from ventral branches of the dorsal aorta, specifically the vitelline arteries.

50–C. The superior mesenteric artery is derived from ventral branches of the dorsal aorta, specifically the vitelline arteries.

51–C. The internal iliac arteries are derived from the ventral branches of the dorsal aorta, specifically the umbilical arteries.

52–A. Arteries to the upper extremity are derived from posterolateral branches of the dorsal aorta.

53–B. The gonadal arteries are derived from lateral branches of the dorsal aorta.

54–C. The proximal part of the internal carotid artery is derived from aortic arch 3.

55–D. Part of the arch of the aorta is derived from aortic arch 4.

56–B. The stapedial artery is derived from aortic arch 2.

57–F. The proximal part of the left pulmonary artery is derived from aortic arch 6.

58–D. The proximal part of the right subclavian artery is derived from aortic arch 4.

59–C. The common carotid arteries are derived from aortic arch 3.

60–F. The proximal part of the right pulmonary artery is derived from aortic arch 6.

61–A. The portal vein is derived from the right vitelline vein.

62–C. The internal jugular veins are derived from the anterior cardinal veins.

63–F. The azygos vein is derived from the supracardinal veins.

64–E. The renal veins are derived from the subcardinal veins.

65–C. The superior vena cava is derived from the right anterior cardinal vein.

66–F. The hemiazygos vein is derived from the supracardinal veins.

67–A. The superior mesenteric vein is derived from the vitelline veins.

68–D. The common iliac veins are derived from the posterior cardinal veins.

6

Placenta and Amniotic Fluid

I. Formation of the Placenta (Figure 6-1)

- The placenta is formed as the endometrium of the uterus is invaded by the developing embryo and as the trophoblast forms the villous chorion.
- Villous chorion formation goes through three stages: **primary chorionic villi, secondary chorionic villi,** and **tertiary chorionic villi**.

II. Placental Components: Decidua Basalis and Villous Chorion (Figure 6-2)

A. Maternal component

1. This consists structurally of the **decidua basalis**, which is derived from the endometrium of the uterus located between the blastocyst and the myometrium.

2. The decidua basalis and **decidua parietalis** (which includes all portions of the endometrium other than the site of implantation) are shed as part of the afterbirth.

3. The **decidua capsularis**, the portion of endometrium that covers the blastocyst and separates it from the uterine cavity, becomes attenuated and degenerates at week 22 of development because of a reduced blood supply.

4. The term decidua means "falling off," "shed," or "sloughed off."

B. Fetal component

- consists of tertiary chorionic villi derived from both the trophoblast and extraembryonic mesoderm, which collectively become known as the **villous chorion**.

1. The villous chorion develops most prolifically at the site of the decidua basalis.

2. The villous chorion is in contrast to an area of no villus development known as the **smooth chorion** (which is related to the decidua capsularis).

III. Appearance of the Placenta in Afterbirth

A. Maternal surface of placenta

65

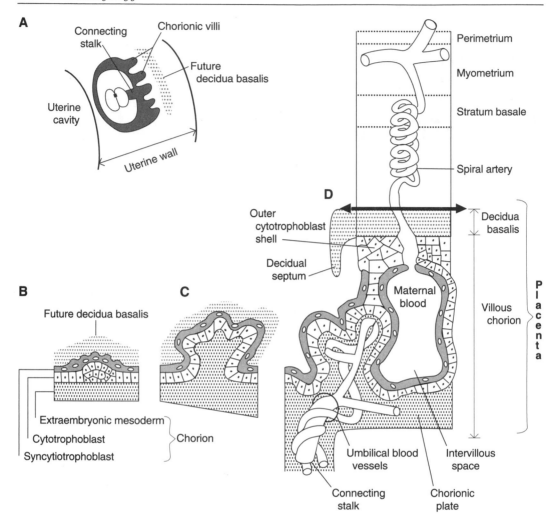

Figure 6-1. Diagram of the various stages of villous chorion formation as it relates to placental development. *(A)* A week 2 embryo completely embedded in the wall of the uterus. *(B)* Primary chorionic villus during week 2 of development. *(C)* Secondary chorionic villus during the start of week 3. *(D)* Tertiary chorionic villus at the end of week 3. The villous chorion and decidua basalis are the two components of the definitive placenta. Note that the cytotrophoblast penetrates the syncytiotrophoblast to make contact with the decidua basalis and form the outer cytotrophoblast shell. The thick double-headed arrow indicates the plane of separation when the placenta is shed during the afterbirth. (Note: The stratum basale is not part of the placenta.)

    – is characterized by 15 to 20 compartments called **cotyledons**, which are
      separated by decidual (placental) septa.
    – is dark red in color.
    – oozes blood due to torn maternal blood vessels.

B. Fetal surface of placenta
    – is characterized by the well-vascularized chorionic plate containing the chori-
      onic blood vessels.
    – has a smooth and shiny appearance because of the amnion.

IV. Functions of the Placenta

A. Metabolism

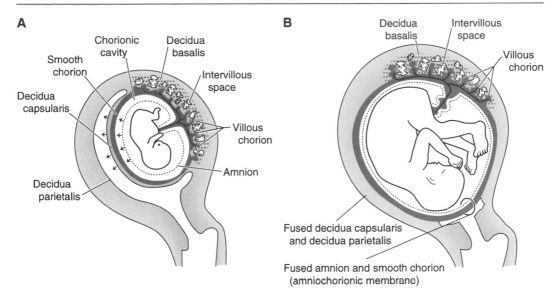

Figure 6-2. Diagram showing the relationship of the fetus, uterus, and placenta. *(A)* Early fetal period. The small arrows (outer set) indicate that as the fetus grows within the uterine wall the decidua capsularis expands and fuses with the decidua parietalis, thereby obliterating the uterine cavity. The small arrows (inner set) indicate that as the fetus grows, the amnion expands toward the smooth chorion, thereby obliterating the chorionic cavity. *(B)* Late fetal period. The uterine cavity and chorionic cavity are obliterated. The fused amnion and smooth chorion form the amniochorionic membrane ("bag of waters"), which passes over the cervical opening.

- The placenta synthesizes and metabolizes glycogen, cholesterol, and fatty acids as a source of nutrients for the fetus.

B. Transport
- The placenta transports a wide variety of substances via diffusion, facilitated diffusion, active transport, and pinocytosis.
- This allows for excretion of waste products by the fetus.

C. Hormone production
- The placenta synthesizes human chorionic gonadotropin (hCG), human placental lactogen (hPL), human chorionic thyrotropin (hCT), human chorionic adrenocorticotropin (hACT), prolactin, relaxin, prostaglandins, progesterone, and estrogen.

V. Placental Membrane (Figure 6-3)
– separates maternal blood from fetal blood.

A. Layers

1. The placenta has four layers in early pregnancy: **syncytiotrophoblast, cytotrophoblast (Langhans cells), connective tissue,** and **endothelium of fetal capillaries**. Hofbauer cells, large elliptical cells found in the connective tissue, are most numerous in early pregnancy; they have characteristics similar to those of macrophages.

2. The placenta has two layers in late pregnancy: **syncytiotrophoblast** and **endothelium of fetal capillaries**.

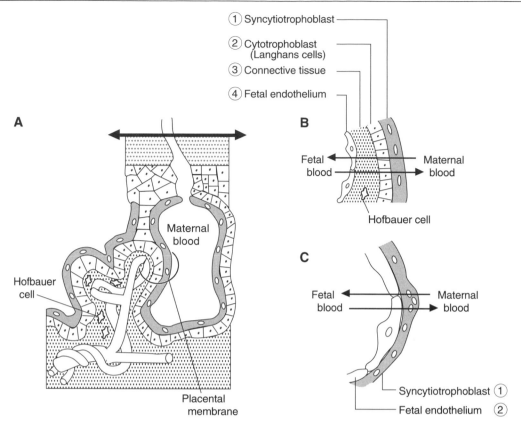

Figure 6-3. Diagram of the placental membrane at *(A and B)* early pregnancy and *(C)* late pregnancy. Langhans' cells are cytotrophoblastic cells that serve as stem cells for the syncytiotrophoblast.

B. Function

- A common misperception is that the placental membrane acts as a strict "barrier." However, a wide variety of substances freely cross the placental membrane.
- Both beneficial and harmful substances can cross the placental membrane (Table 6-1).
- Some substances do not cross the placental membrane (Table 6-1).

VI. Umbilical Cord

A. A patent opening called the **primitive umbilical ring** exists on the ventral surface of the developing embryo.

B. Three structures pass through the primitive umbilical ring: **yolk sac (vitelline duct), connecting stalk,** and **allantois**.

- The allantois is not functional in humans and degenerates to form the **median umbilical ligament** in the adult.

C. As the amnion expands, it pushes the vitelline duct, connecting stalk, and allantois together to form the **primitive umbilical cord**.

Table 6-1. Substances That Cross or Do Not Cross the Placental Membrane

Substances That Cross the Placental Membrane

Beneficial Substances

Gases: Oxygen, carbon dioxide

Nutrients: Glucose, amino acids, free fatty acids, vitamins

Electrolytes: Water, sodium, potassium chloride, calcium phosphate

Fetal waste products: Carbon dioxide, urea, uric acid, bilirubin

Cells: Fetal and maternal red blood cells

Proteins: Maternal serum proteins*

Harmful Substances

Gases: Carbon monoxide

Viruses: Human immunodeficiency virus (HIV), cytomegalovirus, rubella, coxsackievirus, variola, varicella, measles, poliomyelitis

Immunoglobulins: IgG (anti-Rh antibodies)

Drugs: Thalidomide, cocaine, alcohol, caffeine, nicotine, warfarin, trimethadione, phenytoin, cancer chemo agents, anesthetics, sedatives, analgesics†

Microorganisms: Treponema pallidum, Toxoplasma gondii

Substances That Do NOT Cross the Placental Membrane

Nutrients: Maternally derived cholesterol, triglycerides, phospholipids

Hormones: All protein hormones (including insulin)

Immunoglobulins: IgM

Drugs: Succinylcholine, curare, heparin, drugs similar to amino acids (methyldopa)

Microorganisms: Bacteria

* Cross at a very low rate; most fetal serum proteins are synthesized de novo by the fetus.
† In general, most drugs and their metabolites cross the placental membrane.

    D. At week 6 of development, the gut tube connected to the yolk sac will herniate **(physiological umbilical herniation)** into the extraembryonic coelom; the herniation will be reduced by week 11.

    E. The gut tube eventually returns to the abdominal cavity; the yolk sac (vitelline duct) and allantois degenerate.

    F. The definitive umbilical cord contains the **right and left umbilical arteries, left umbilical vein,** and **mucus connective tissue (Wharton's jelly)**.

VII. Circulatory System of the Fetus (Figure 6-4)

    – Fetal circulation involves three shunts: the **ductus venosus, ductus arteriosus,** and **foramen ovale**.

    A. Highly oxygenated and nutrient-enriched blood returns to the fetus from the placenta via the **left umbilical vein**. (Note: Highly oxygenated blood is carried by the left umbilical vein, not by an artery as in the adult.)

        1. Some blood percolates through the hepatic sinusoids; most of the blood bypasses the sinusoids by passing through the ductus venosus and enters the inferior vena cava.

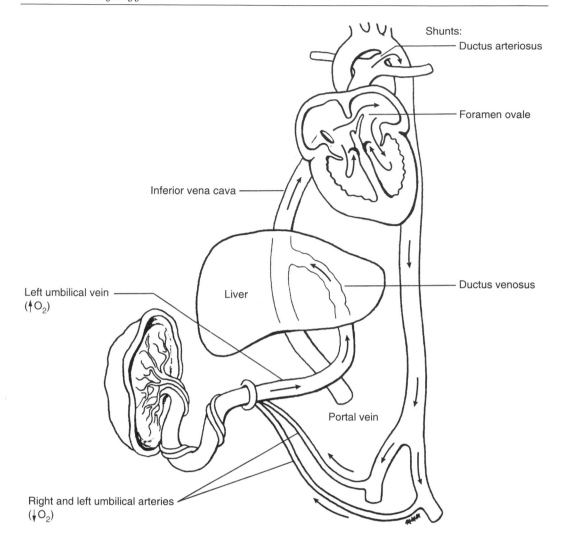

Figure 6-4. Schematic diagram of fetal circulation. (Reprinted from Dudek RW: *High-Yield Embryology.* Baltimore, Williams & Wilkins, 1996, p. 14.)

2. From the inferior vena cava, blood enters the right atrium, where most of the blood bypasses the right ventricle through the foramen ovale to enter the left atrium.

3. From the left atrium, blood enters the left ventricle and is delivered to fetal tissues via the aorta.

B. Poorly oxygenated and nutrient-poor fetal blood is sent back to the placenta via **right and left umbilical arteries**.

C. Some blood in the right atrium enters the right ventricle; blood in the right ventricle enters the pulmonary trunk, but most of the blood bypasses the lungs through the **ductus arteriosus**.

1. Fetal lungs receive only a minimal amount of blood for growth and development; the blood is returned to the left ventricle via pulmonary veins.

2. Fetal lungs are not capable of performing their adult respiratory function because they are functionally immature and the fetus is underwater (amniotic fluid). The placenta provides respiratory function.

D. Circulatory system changes at birth are facilitated by a decrease in right atrial pressure from occlusion of placental circulation and by an increase in left atrial pressure due to increased pulmonary venous return.

– Changes include closure of:

1. umbilical arteries

2. umbilical vein

3. ductus venosus

4. ductus arteriosus

5. foramen ovale

VIII. Amniotic Fluid

A. Components

– Amniotic fluid is basically water that contains carbohydrates, lipids, proteins (hormones, enzymes, alpha-fetoprotein), desquamated fetal cells, and fetal urine.

B. Production

– Amniotic fluid is constantly produced during pregnancy by the following:

1. Dialysis of maternal blood through blood vessels in the placenta

2. Dialysis of fetal blood through blood vessels in the placenta and umbilical cord

3. Excretion of fetal urine into the amniotic sac

C. Resorption

– Amniotic fluid is constantly resorbed during pregnancy by several possible routes, one of which is the following sequence of events:

1. Fetus swallows amniotic fluid.

2. Amniotic fluid is absorbed into the fetal blood stream through the gastrointestinal tract.

3. Excess amniotic fluid is removed via the placenta into the maternal blood stream.

D. Amount of amniotic fluid

– is gradually increased during pregnancy from **50 ml at week 12** of development to **1000 ml at term**.

– The rate of water exchange within the amniotic sac at term is 400–500 ml/hr, with a net flow of 125–200 ml/hr moving from the amniotic fluid into the maternal blood stream.

– The near-term fetus excretes about 500 ml of urine daily, which is mostly water because the placenta exchanges metabolic wastes. The fetus swallows about 400 ml of amniotic fluid daily.

IX. Clinical Considerations

A. Complete hydatidiform mole

– is a blighted blastocyst (embryo dies), which is retained in the uterine wall, followed by hyperplastic proliferation of the trophoblast and cystic swelling.
– Cysts (like bunches of grapes) form and fill the uterine cavity.
– Diagnostic aids include ultrasound, continued rise of hCG levels, and development of preeclampsia (a combination of hypertension and proteinuria).
– Karyotyping has indicated that complete moles consist of chromosomes derived entirely from the father.

B. Choriocarcinoma

– is a malignant tumor of the trophoblast.
– presents clinically as repeated uterine bleeding.
– may occur following a normal pregnancy, abortion, or hydatidiform mole.
– is associated with high hCG levels.
– metastasizes via the blood stream.

C. Premature rupture of the amniochorionic membrane

– is the most common cause of premature labor and oligohydramnios.
– is commonly referred to as "breaking of the waters."

D. Amniotic band syndrome

– occurs when bands of amniotic membrane encircle and constrict various parts of the fetus, causing limb and craniofacial anomalies.

E. Presence of one umbilical artery within the cord

– is an abnormal condition that generally indicates the presence of cardiovascular anomalies. (Normally two umbilical arteries are present.)

F. Abnormal placental shapes

1. Velamentous placenta

– is a placenta in which the umbilical vessels travel abnormally through the amniochorionic membrane before reaching the placenta proper.
– If the umbilical vessels cross the internal os, a serious condition called vasa previa exists. In vasa previa, if one of the umbilical vessels ruptures during pregnancy, labor, or delivery, the fetus will bleed to death.

2. Bipartite or tripartite placenta

– is a placenta made up of two or three connected lobes.

3. Duplex or triplex placenta

– is a placenta made up of two or three separate lobes.

4. Succenturiate placenta

– is a placenta consisting of small accessory lobes completely separate from the main placenta.

– Care must be taken to assure that the accessory lobes are eliminated in the afterbirth.

5. Membranous placenta

– is a thin placenta that forms over the greater part of the uterine cavity.
– Care must be taken to assure that all the placenta is eliminated during the afterbirth; may require curettage.

G. Placenta previa

– occurs when the placenta attaches in the lower part of the uterus, covering the internal os. (The placenta normally implants in the posterior superior wall of the uterus.)
– Uterine vessels rupture during the later part of pregnancy as the uterus begins to gradually dilate.
– The mother may bleed to death, and the fetus will also be placed in jeopardy because of the compromised blood supply.
– Because the placenta blocks the cervical opening, delivery is usually accomplished by cesarean section.
– is clinically associated with repeated episodes of bright red vaginal bleeding.

H. Placental abruption

– occurs when a normally implanted placenta prematurely separates from the uterus before delivery of the fetus.
– is associated with maternal hypertension.

I. Erythroblastosis fetalis

– occurs when Rh-positive fetal red blood cells (RBCs) cross the placental membrane into the maternal circulation of an Rh-negative mother; the mother forms anti-Rh antibodies that cross the placental membrane and destroy fetal RBCs.
– Destruction of fetal RBCs releases large amounts of bilirubin, leading to cerebral damage and sometimes death of the fetus.

J. Oligohydramnios

– is a low amount of amniotic fluid, about **400 ml in late pregnancy**.
– results in fetal deformities (Potter's syndrome) and possibly hypoplastic lungs due to increased pressure on the fetus.
– may be associated with failure of the fetus to excrete urine into the amniotic fluid due to renal agenesis.

K. Polyhydramnios

– is a high amount of amniotic fluid, about **2000 ml in late pregnancy**.
– is clinically associated with anencephaly or esophageal atresia, both of which impair the ability of the fetus to swallow.
– is commonly associated with maternal diabetes.

L. Twinning

1. Monozygotic (identical) twins develop from one zygote and in 65% of the cases have **one placenta, one chorion,** and **two amniotic sacs**.

    2. Dizygotic (fraternal) twins develop from two zygotes and have **two placentas, two chorions,** and **two amniotic sacs**.

M. Alpha-fetoprotein (AFP)
- is found in amniotic fluid and maternal serum.
- Elevated levels are a good indicator of neural tube defects.
- Reduced levels may be associated with Down's Syndrome.

Review Test

Directions: Each of the numbered items or incomplete statements in this section is followed by answers or by completions of the statement. Select the **one** lettered answer or completion that is **best** in each case.

1. During the later stages of pregnancy, maternal blood is separated from fetal blood by the

(A) syncytiotrophoblast only
(B) cytotrophoblast only
(C) syncytiotrophoblast and cytotrophoblast
(D) syncytiotrophoblast and fetal endothelium
(E) cytotrophoblast and fetal endothelium

2. The maternal and fetal components of the placenta are

(A) decidua basalis and secondary chorionic villi
(B) decidua capsularis and secondary chorionic villi
(C) decidua parietalis and tertiary chorionic villi
(D) decidua capsularis and villous chorion
(E) decidua basalis and villous chorion

3. The intervillous space of the placenta contains

(A) maternal blood
(B) fetal blood
(C) maternal and fetal blood
(D) amniotic fluid
(E) maternal blood and amniotic fluid

4. A young insulin-dependent diabetic woman in her first pregnancy is concerned that her daily injection of insulin will cause a congenital malformation in her baby. What should the physician tell her?

(A) Insulin is highly teratogenic; discontinue treatment
(B) Insulin does not cross the placental membrane
(C) Insulin crosses the placental membrane but is degraded rapidly
(D) Insulin will benefit her baby by increasing glucose metabolism
(E) Insulin crosses the placental membrane but is not teratogenic

5. What is a normal amount of amniotic fluid at term?

(A) 50 ml
(B) 500 ml
(C) 1000 ml
(D) 1500 ml
(E) 2000 ml

6. All of the following pass through the primitive umbilical ring EXCEPT

(A) allantois
(B) amnion
(C) yolk sac
(D) connecting stalk
(E) space connecting the intraembryonic and extraembryonic coeloms

7. A 42-year-old woman presents with complaints of severe headaches, blurred vision, slurred speech, and loss of muscle coordination. Her last pregnancy 5 years ago resulted in a hydatidiform mole. Laboratory results show a high hCG level. Which of the following conditions is a probable diagnosis?

(A) Vasa previa
(B) Placenta previa
(C) Succenturiate placenta
(D) Choriocarcinoma
(E) Membranous placenta

8. A 26-year-old pregnant woman experiences repeated episodes of bright red vaginal bleeding at week 28, week 32, and week 34 of pregnancy. The bleeding spontaneously subsided each time. Using ultrasound, the placenta is located in the lower right portion of the uterus over the internal os. What is the diagnosis?

(A) Hydatidiform mole
(B) Vasa previa
(C) Placenta previa
(D) Placental abruption
(E) Premature rupture of the amniochorionic membrane

9. A 19-year-old woman in week 32 of a complication-free pregnancy is rushed to the emergency department because of profuse vaginal bleeding. The bleeding subsides, but afterwards no fetal heart sounds can be heard, indicating intrauterine fetal death. The woman goes into labor and delivers a stillborn infant. On examination of the afterbirth, a velamentous placenta is detected. Although not much can be done at this point, what is the diagnosis?

(A) Placenta previa
(B) Vasa previa
(C) Hydatidiform mole
(D) Premature rupture of the amniochorionic membrane
(E) Amniotic band syndrome

Directions: Each group of items in this section consists of lettered options followed by a set of numbered items. For each item, select the **one** lettered option that is most closely associated with it. Each lettered option may be selected once, more than once, or not at all.

Questions 10–20

Match the substances below with the appropriate action.

(A) Crosses the placental membrane
(B) Does not cross the placental membrane

10. Steroid hormones

11. Immunoglobulin G (IgG)

12. Bacteria

13. Fetal red blood cells (RBCs)

14. Protein hormones

15. Glucose

16. Human immunodeficiency virus

17. Succinylcholine

18. Maternal cholesterol

19. Cocaine

20. Methyldopa

Answers and Explanations

1–D. During the later stages of pregnancy, the placental membrane becomes very thin and consists of two layers, the syncytiotrophoblast and fetal endothelium.

2–E. The placenta is a unique organ in that it is a composite of tissue from two different sources, the mother and fetus. The maternal component is the decidua basalis, and the fetal component is the villous chorion.

3–A. The intervillous space contains only maternal blood because the spiral arteries of the endometrium penetrate the outer cytotrophoblast shell.

4–B. Insulin, like all protein hormones, does not cross the placental membrane in significant amounts.

5–C. The normal amount of amniotic fluid at term is 1000 ml. However, the amount of amniotic fluid at various stages of pregnancy can be indicative of congenital malformations. Oligohydramnios (400 ml in late pregnancy) may be indicative of renal agenesis. Polyhydramnios (2000 ml in late pregnancy) may be indicative of either anencephaly or esophageal atresia.

6–B. The amnion does not pass through the primitive umbilical ring. As craniocaudal folding occurs, the amnion becomes the outer covering of the umbilical cord.

7–D. After a hydatidiform mole, it is very important to assure that all the invasive trophoblastic tissue is removed. High levels of hCG are a good indicator of retained trophoblastic tissue because such tissue produces this hormone. In this case, the trophoblastic tissue has developed into a malignant choriocarcinoma and metastasized to the brain, causing her symptoms of headache, blurred vision, and so on.

8–C. A placenta implanted in the lower part of the uterus near the internal os is called placenta previa. The repeated episodes of bright red vaginal bleeding are caused by the gradual dilation of the uterus in the later stages of pregnancy. As the uterus dilates, spiral arteries and veins supplying the placenta are ruptured. The mother may bleed to death, and the fetus is placed in jeopardy because of the compromised maternal blood flow.

9–B. A velamentous placenta occurs when umbilical blood vessels abnormally travel through the amniochorionic membrane before reaching the placenta proper. If the vessels cross the internal os, a serious condition called vasa previa exists. As the fetus grows during pregnancy and the amniochorionic membrane stretches, the umbilical vessels may rupture. When that happens, the fetus will bleed to death. The mother is in no danger of bleeding to death in vasa previa because only the umbilical vessels rupture.

10–A. Unconjugated steroid hormones cross the placental membrane freely. Testosterone and synthetic progestins cross the placental membrane and cause masculinization in female fetuses.

11–A. Maternal IgG crosses the placental membrane and imparts fetal immunity to such diseases as diphtheria, smallpox, and measles. In some cases, maternal IgG may have a harmful effect on the fetus, as in erythroblastosis fetalis (anti-Rh antibodies).

12–B. Bacteria are generally considered not to cross the placental membrane. However, bacterial infections can cause lesions in the placental membrane, which then allow bacteria to cross through the "breaks" in the placental membrane.

13–A. Small amounts of maternal and fetal blood may cross through small "breaks" in the placental membrane. The crossing of fetal RBCs into the maternal circulation is important in the etiology of erythroblastosis fetalis.

14–B. Protein hormones (such as insulin) do not cross the placental membrane in significant amounts.

15–A. Glucose freely crosses the placental membrane. In maternal diabetes, exposure of the fetus to high levels of glucose may result in fetal macrosomia.

16–A. Viruses cross the placental membrane and can seriously affect the fetus.

17–B. Although most drugs cross the placental membrane, succinylcholine does not.

18–B. Maternal cholesterol, triglycerides, and phospholipids do not cross the placental membrane.

19–A. Cocaine crosses the placental membrane and causes a physiologic addiction in the fetus.

20–B. Drugs that have a structural similarity to amino acids do not cross the placental membrane even though amino acids (nutrients) do cross.

7
Nervous System

I. Overview

A. Central nervous system (CNS)
- is formed in week 3 of development as the **neural plate**.
- The neural plate consisting of **neuroectoderm** becomes the **neural tube**, which gives rise to the brain and spinal cord.

B. Peripheral nervous system (PNS)
- is derived from three sources:

  1. **Neural crest cells** give rise to peripheral ganglia, Schwann cells, and afferent nerve fibers (from dorsal root ganglia).

  2. **Neural tube** gives rise to all preganglionic autonomic fibers and all fibers that innervate skeletal muscles.

  3. **Mesoderm** gives rise to the dura mater and to connective tissue investments of peripheral nerve fibers (endoneurium, perineurium, and epineurium).

II. Development of the Neural Tube (Figure 7-1)
- begins in week 3 due to the inductive influence of the **notochord,** which directs **surface ectoderm** to differentiate into neuroectoderm and is completed in week 4.

A. Neural plate
- is a thickened pear-shaped region of neuroectoderm, located between the primitive knot and the oropharyngeal membrane.

B. Neural groove
- forms as the neural plate begins to fold inward.
- is flanked by parallel neural folds.

C. Neural folds
- fuse in the midline to form the neural tube.
- are the sites of **neural crest differentiation**.

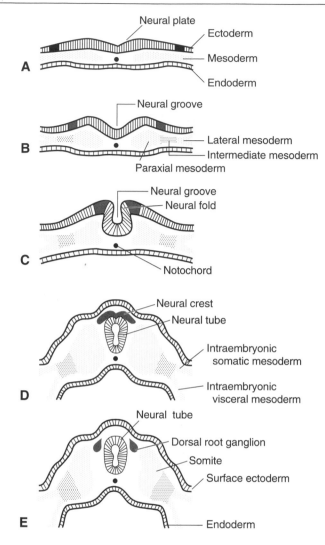

Figure 7-1. Schematic diagrams of transverse sections of embryos at various stages. *(A)* Neural plate stage. *(B)* Early neural groove stage. *(C)* Late neural groove stage. *(D)* Early neural tube and neural crest stage. *(E)* Neural tube and dorsal root ganglion stage. (Modified from Truex RC and Carpenter MB: *Human Neuroanatomy.* Baltimore, Williams & Wilkins, 1969, p. 91.)

D. Neural tube

— forms as the neural folds fuse in the midline and separate from the surface ectoderm.

— gives rise to the CNS:

1. The cranial part becomes the brain.

2. The caudal part becomes the spinal cord.

3. The lumen gives rise to the central canal of the spinal cord and the ventricles of the brain.

4. The **anterior and posterior neuropores** connect the central canal with the amniotic cavity.

  a. **Anterior neuropore** closes during week 4 (day 25) and becomes the **lamina terminalis**.
    – Failure of the anterior neuropore to close results in **anencephaly**.

  b. **Posterior neuropore** closes during week 4 (day 27).
    – Failure of the posterior neuropore to close results in **spina bifida**.

III. Neural Crest (see Figure 7-1)
– See Table 4-1.

IV. Placodes
– are localized thickenings of surface **ectoderm**.
– give rise to cells that migrate into underlying mesoderm and develop into sensory receptive organs of cranial nerves (CN I and CN VIII) and the lens of the eye.

A. Lens placode
– gives rise to the **lens**.
– is induced by the optic vesicles.

B. Nasal (olfactory) placodes
– differentiate into neurosensory cells that give rise to the **olfactory nerve (CN I)**.
– induce formation of olfactory bulbs.

C. Otic placodes
– give rise to the **otic vesicle,** which forms the:

  1. Utricle, semicircular ducts, and vestibular ganglion of CN VIII

  2. Saccule, cochlear duct (organ of Corti), spiral ganglion of CN VIII

  3. Vestibulocochlear nerve (CN VIII)

V. Stages of Neural Tube Development

A. Vesicle development

  1. The three **primary brain vesicles** and two associated flexures develop during week 4 (Figures 7-2A and 7-2B).

    a. **Prosencephalon (forebrain)**
      – is associated with the appearance of the **optic vesicles**.
      – gives rise to the telencephalon (endbrain) and the diencephalon (betweenbrain).

    b. **Mesencephalon (midbrain)**
      – remains as the mesencephalon.

    c. **Rhombencephalon (hindbrain)**
      – gives rise to the metencephalon (afterbrain), which forms the pons and the cerebellum, and the myelencephalon (medulla oblongata).

    d. **Cephalic flexure (midbrain flexure)**
      – is located between the prosencephalon and the rhombencephalon.

    e. **Cervical flexure**
      – is located between the rhombencephalon and the future spinal cord.

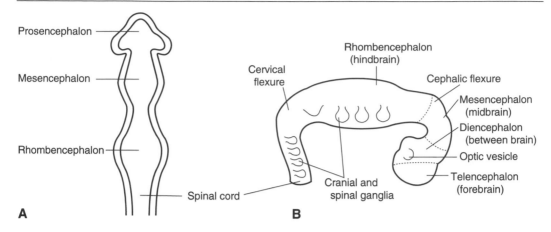

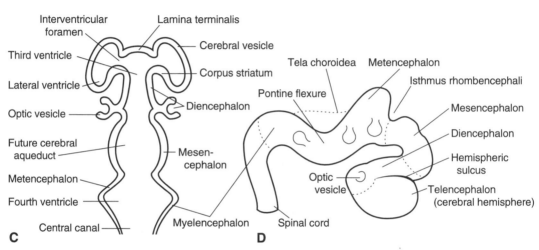

Figure 7-2. Schematic illustrations of the developing brain vesicles and ventricular system. *(A and B)* Three-brain-vesicle stage of a 4-week-old embryo. *(C and D)* Five-brain-vesicle stage of a 6-week-old embryo. (Modified from Truex RC and Carpenter MB: *Human Neuroanatomy.* Baltimore, Williams & Wilkins, 1969, p. 97.)

    2. Five **secondary brain vesicles** (Figures 7-2*C* and 7-2*D*) become visible in week 6 of development and form various adult derivatives of the brain (Table 7-1).

B. Histogenesis

    1. Cells of the neural tube wall

       – are neuroectodermal (or neuroepithelial) cells that give rise to the following:

      a. Neuroblasts

         – form all neurons found in the CNS.

      b. Glioblasts (spongioblasts)

         – are, for the most part, formed after cessation of neuroblast formation. Radial glial cells are an exception and develop before neurogenesis is complete.

         – form the supporting cells of the CNS.

Table 7-1. Primary and Secondary Embryonic Vesicles and Their Adult Derivatives

Primary Vesicles	Secondary Vesicles	Adult Derivatives
Prosencephalon	Telencephalon	Cerebral hemispheres, caudate, putamen, amygdaloid, claustrum, lamina terminalis, olfactory bulbs, hippocampus
	Diencephalon	Epithalamus, pineal gland, thalamus, hypothalamus, mammillary bodies, neurohypophysis, subthalamus, globus pallidus, retina, iris, ciliary body, optic nerve (CN II), optic chiasm, optic tract
Mesencephalon	Mesencephalon	Midbrain
Rhombencephalon	Metencephalon	Pons, cerebellum
	Myelencephalon	Medulla

(1) **Macroglia**

(a) **Astroglia (astrocytes)**
- contain **glial fibrillary acitic protein (GFAP)**, a marker for astroblasts.
- surround blood capillaries with their vascular feet.

(b) **Radial glial cells**
- are of astrocytic lineage and are GFAP-positive.
- provide guidance for migrating neuroblasts.

(c) **Oligodendroglia (oligodendrocytes)**
- produce the **myelin** of the CNS.

(2) **Ependymal cells**

(a) **Ependymocytes**
- line the ventricles and the central canal.

(b) **Tanycytes**
- are located in the wall of the third ventricle.
- transport substances from the cerebrospinal fluid (CSF) to the hypophyseal portal system.

(c) **Choroid plexus cells**
- produce **CSF**.
- are bound together by tight junctions that represent the blood–CSF barrier.

c. **Microglia (Hortega cells)**
- are the scavenger cells of the CNS.
- arise from monocytes.
- invade the developing nervous system in week 3 with the developing blood vessels.

2. **Layers of the early neural tube wall**

a. **Spinal cord**

(1) **Ventricular zone (neuroepithelial layer)**
- gives rise to a layer of ependymal cells, which line the central canal.

- cells migrate into the intermediate layer.
- gives rise to all neurons and glial cells of the spinal cord.

(2) **Intermediate zone (mantle layer)**

- consists of neurons and glial cells of the **gray matter of the spinal cord**.
- contains the developing alar and basal plates.

(3) **Marginal zone**

- contains nerve fibers (axons) of the neuroblasts of the mantle layer and glial cells.
- **forms the white matter of the spinal cord** through myelination of axons.

b. **Brain**

(1) **Ventricular zone (neuroepithelial layer)**

- gives rise to a layer of ependymal cells, which line the ventricles.
- gives rise to all **neurons and glial cells of the brain**.

(2) **Intermediate zone (mantle layer)**

- with the ventricular layer, gives rise to the **cerebral cortex** and **basal ganglia**.

(3) **Marginal zone**

- becomes the molecular layer of the cortex, which underlies the pia.

(4) **Cortex**

- is the **gray matter** of the cerebral hemispheres.

VI. Development of the Spinal Cord (Figure 7-3)

- The spinal cord develops from the neural tube caudal to the fourth pair of somites.

A. **Neural tube components**

1. **Alar plate**

   - is a **dorsolateral** thickening of the intermediate zone (mantle layer) of the neural tube.
   - gives rise to **sensory neuroblasts of the dorsal horn** (general somatic afferent [GSA] and general visceral afferent [GVA] cell regions).
   - receives axons, which become the dorsal roots, from the dorsal root ganglion.
   - becomes the **dorsal horn of the spinal cord**.

2. **Basal plate**

   - is a **ventrolateral** thickening of the intermediate zone (mantle layer) of the neural tube.
   - gives rise to **motor neuroblasts of the ventral and lateral horns** (general somatic efferent [GSE] and general visceral efferent [GVE] cell regions).
   - Axons from motor neuroblasts exit the spinal cord and form the ventral roots.
   - becomes the **ventral horn of the spinal cord**.

3. **Sulcus limitans**

   - is a **longitudinal groove** in the lateral wall of the neural tube that appears during week 4 of development.

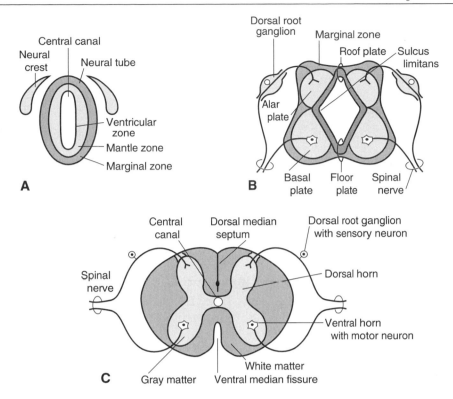

Figure 7-3. Schematic illustration of three successive stages in the development of the spinal cord. Note that the neural crest gives rise to the dorsal root ganglion and that the alar and basal plates give rise to the dorsal and ventral horns, respectively.

- separates the alar (sensory) and basal (motor) plates.
- disappears in the adult spinal cord, but is retained in the rhomboid fossa of the brain stem.
- extends from the spinal cord to the rostral midbrain.

4. Roof plate

- is the nonneural roof of the central canal, which connects the two alar plates.

5. Floor plate

- is the nonneural floor of the central canal, which connects the two basal plates.
- contains the ventral white commissure.

6. Caudal eminence

- arises from the primitive streak.
- blends with the neural tube and gives rise to caudal **sacral and coccygeal segments of the spinal cord**.

B. Myelination

- begins during month 4 in the spinal cord motor roots.

1. Oligodendrocytes accomplish myelination of the **CNS**.

2. Schwann cells accomplish myelination of the **PNS**.

3. Myelination of the corticospinal tracts is not completed until the end of 2 years of age (i.e., when the corticospinal tracts become myelinated and functional).

4. Myelination of the **association neocortex** extends to 30 years of age.

C. Positional changes of the spinal cord

- At week 8 of development, the spinal cord extends the length of the vertebral canal.
- At birth, the **conus medullaris** extends to the level of the third lumbar vertebra (**L-3**).
- In adults, the conus medullaris terminates at **L1–L2 interspace**.
- Disparate growth (between the vertebral column and the spinal cord) results in the formation of the **cauda equina**, consisting of dorsal and ventral roots, which descends below the level of the conus medullaris.
- Disparate growth results in the nonneural **filum terminale**, which anchors the spinal cord to the coccyx.

VII. Development of Myelencephalon (Figures 7-4 and 7-5)

- The myelencephalon develops from the **rhombencephalon**.
- It gives rise to the **medulla oblongata**.

A. Alar (sensory) and basal (motor) plates

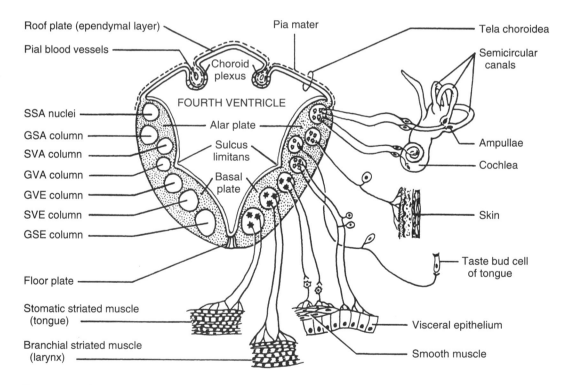

Figure 7-4. Schematic diagram of the brain stem, illustrating the cell columns derived from alar and basal plates. The seven cranial nerve modalities are shown. *GSA* = general somatic afferent; *GSE* = general somatic efferent; *GVA* = general visceral afferent; *GVE* = general visceral efferent; *SSA* = special somatic afferent; *SVA* = special visceral afferent; *SVE* = special visceral efferent. (Modified from Patten BM: *Human Embryology,* 3rd ed. New York, The Blakiston Division, McGraw-Hill, 1969, p. 298.)

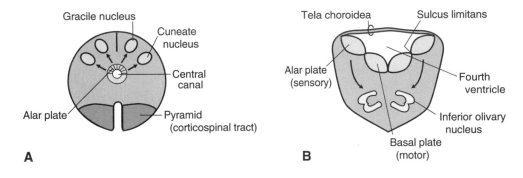

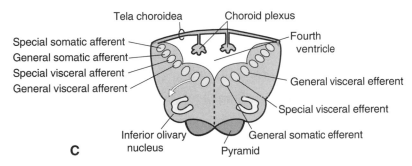

Figure 7-5. Schematic illustrations of the development of the medulla. *(A)* Transverse section of the caudal medulla, showing the development of the gracile and cuneate nuclei from the alar plates. *(B)* Schematic sketch through the rostral (open) medulla, showing the relationships of the alar and basal plates; the inferior olivary nucleus is derived from the alar plate. *(C)* A later stage of B shows the four sensory modalities of the alar plate and the three motor modalities of the basal plate; the white arrow indicates the lateral migration of the special visceral efferent (SVE) column (CN IX, X, and XI); pyramids consist of motor fibers, the corticospinal tracts.

1. **Alar plate sensory neuroblasts** give rise to the following:

   a. **Dorsal column nuclei**, which consist of the gracile and cuneate nuclei

   b. **Inferior olivary nuclei**, which are cerebellar relay nuclei

   c. **Solitary nucleus**, which forms the general visceral afferent (GVA) [taste] and special visceral afferent (SVA) column

   d. **Spinal trigeminal nucleus**, which forms the general somatic afferent (GSA) column

   e. **Cochlear and vestibular nuclei**
      – form the special somatic afferent (SSA) column.
      – lie in the medullopontine junction.

2. **Basal plate motor neuroblasts** give rise to the following:

   a. **Hypoglossal nucleus**, which forms the general somatic efferent (GSE) column

   b. **Nucleus ambiguus**, which forms the special visceral efferent (SVE) column (CN IX, CN X, and CN XI)

   c. **Dorsal motor nucleus of the vagal nerve (CN X)** and the **inferior salivatory nucleus of the glossopharyngeal nerve (CN IX)**, which form the general visceral efferent (GVE) column

B. Roof plate

- forms the roof of the fourth ventricle.
- is the **tela choroidea**, a monolayer of ependymal cells (lamina epithelialis) covered with pia mater.
- is invaginated by pial vessels to form the **choroid plexus** of the fourth ventricle.

VIII. Development of the Metencephalon (see Figures 7-2C and 7-2D)

- The metencephalon develops from the **rhombencephalon**.
- It gives rise to the **pons** and **cerebellum**.

A. Pons (Figure 7-6)

1. **Alar plate sensory neuroblasts** give rise to the following:

   a. **Solitary nucleus**, which forms the SVA column (taste) of CN VII

   b. **Vestibular and cochlear nuclei**, which form the SSA column of CN VIII

   c. **Spinal and principal trigeminal nuclei**, which form the GSA column of CN V

   d. **Pontine nuclei**, which consist of cerebellar relay nuclei (pontine gray)

2. **Basal plate motor neuroblasts** give rise to the following:

   a. **Abducent nucleus**, which forms the GSE column

   b. **Facial and motor trigeminal nuclei**, which form the SVE column

   c. **Superior salivatory nucleus**, which forms the GVE column of CN VII

3. **Base of pons**
   - contains pontine nuclei from the alar plate.
   - contains corticobulbar, corticospinal, and corticopontine fibers from the cerebral cortex.
   - contains pontocerebellar fibers.

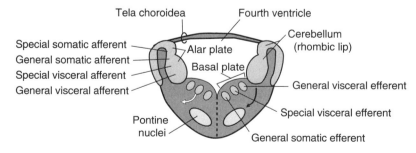

Figure 7-6. Schematic illustration (transverse section) of the development of the pons and cerebellum. The alar plate (rhombic lip) gives rise to the cerebellum, the four sensory cell columns, and the pontine nuclei. The basal plate gives rise to the three motor columns. The base of the pons contains the descending corticospinal tracts, which originate from the motor and sensory strips of the cerebral cortex. The white arrow indicates the lateral migration of the special visceral efferent (SVE) column (CN V and VII).

B. Cerebellum (see Figure 7-6)

– is formed by the **rhombic lips**, which are the two thickened alar plates of the mantle layer.

– New evidence indicates that the rostral part of the cerebellum is derived from the caudal mesencephalon.

– The cerebellar plates give rise to the following:

1. **Vermis**, by midline growth

2. **Cerebellar hemispheres**, by lateral growth

3. **Three-layered cerebellar cortex** (molecular layer, Purkinje cell layer, and [internal] granular layer) and four pairs of cerebellar nuclei, by cell migration from the ventricular zone into the marginal layer

4. **External granular layer (EGL)**

– is a germinal (proliferative) layer on the surface of the cerebellum, present from week 8 of development to 2 years of age.

– New evidence indicates that the EGL gives rise only to granule cells and not to basket (inner stellate) or stellate (outer stellate) neurons, as has been long thought.

– Persistent cell nests may give rise to a neoplasm, medulloblastoma.

– is sensitive to antiviral agents, which block the synthesis of DNA.

5. **Folia and fissures** are formed by differential cortical growth.

IX. Development of the Mesencephalon (Figure 7-7)

– The mesencephalon remains unchanged during primary to secondary vesicle formation.

– It gives rise to the **midbrain.**

A. Alar plate neuroblasts form the cell layers of the **superior colliculi** and the nuclei of the **inferior colliculi.**

B. Basal plate neuroblasts give rise to the following:

1. **Trochlear and oculomotor nuclei of CN IV and CN III**, which form the GSE column

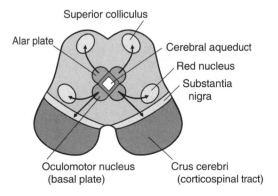

Figure 7-7. Schematic illustration (transverse section) of the development of the midbrain. The alar plate gives rise to the layers of the superior colliculus and to the nuclei of the inferior colliculus. The basal plate gives rise to the oculomotor and trochlear nuclei, the substantia nigra, and the red nucleus. The cerebral peduncles contain the descending corticospinal tracts.

2. **Edinger-Westphal nucleus of CN III**, which forms the most rostral cell group of the GVE column

3. **Substantia nigra**

4. **Red nucleus**

C. **Basis pedunculi (crus cerebri)**
   – contains corticobulbar, corticospinal, and corticopontine fibers, derived from the cerebral cortex of the telencephalon.

X. Development of the Diencephalon, Optic Structures, and Hypophysis

A. **Diencephalon** (Figure 7-8; see also Figure 7-2)
   – The diencephalon develops from the prosencephalon within the walls of the primitive third ventricle.
   – It gives rise to the **epithalamus, thalamus, hypothalamus,** and **subthalamus**.

   1. **Epithalamus**
      – develops from the embryonic roof plate and dorsal parts of alar plates.
      – gives rise to the **pineal body** (epiphysis) and to the **tela choroidea** and choroid plexus of the third ventricle.

   2. **Thalamus**
      – is an alar plate **derivative** that gives rise to the **thalamic nuclei**.

   3. **Hypothalamus**
      – develops from the alar plate and floor plate.
      – gives rise to **hypothalamic nuclei**, including the **mamillary bodies**, and to the **neurohypophysis** (Figure 7-9).

   4. **Subthalamus**
      – is an alar plate derivative.
      – includes the subthalamic nucleus.

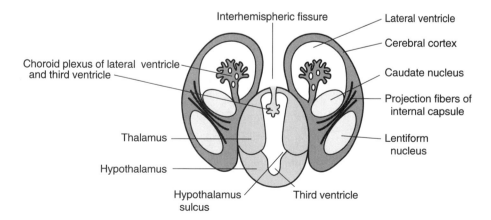

Figure 7-8. Schematic illustration (transverse section) of the development of the forebrain. The cerebral cortex and basal ganglia are shown. The internal capsule divides the corpus striatum into the caudate nucleus and the lentiform nucleus. The alar plate of the diencephalon gives rise to the thalamus and the hypothalamus.

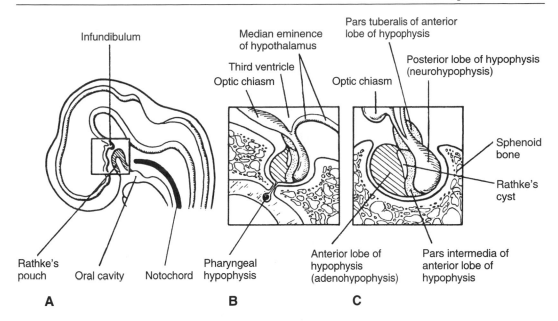

Figure 7-9. Schematic drawings illustrating the development of the hypophysis (pituitary gland). *(A)* Midsagittal section through the 6-week-old embryo, showing Rathke's pouch as a dorsal outpocketing of the oral cavity and the infundibulum as a thickening in the floor of the hypothalamus. *(B and C)* Development at 11 weeks and 16 weeks, respectively. The anterior lobe, the pars tuberalis, and the pars intermedia are derived from Rathke's pouch. (Modified from Sadler TW: *Langman's Medical Embryology,* 6th ed. Baltimore, Williams & Wilkins, 1990, p. 373.)

– gives rise to neuroblasts that migrate into the telencephalic white matter to become the **globus pallidus** (pallidum), a basal ganglion.

B. Optic vesicles, cups, and stalks (see Figure 7-2)

– are derivatives of diencephalon.
– give rise to the **retina, iris, ciliary body, optic nerve (CNII), optic chiasm,** and **optic tract**.

C. Hypophysis (pituitary gland) [see Figure 7-9]

– is attached by the pituitary stalk to the hypothalamus.

1. Anterior lobe (adenohypophysis)

– develops from **Rathke's pouch**, an ectodermal diverticulum of the primitive mouth cavity (stomodeum). Remnants of Rathke's pouch may give rise to a **craniopharyngioma**.

2. Posterior lobe (neurohypophysis)

– develops from a ventral evagination of the hypothalamus.
– includes the median eminence, infundibular stem, and pars nervosa.

XI. Development of the Telencephalon

– The telencephalon develops from the prosencephalon.
– It gives rise to the **cerebral hemispheres, caudate, putamen, amygdaloid, claustrum, lamina terminalis, olfactory bulbs,** and **hippocampus**.

A. Cerebral hemispheres (see Figures 7-2 and 7-8)

- develop as bilateral evaginations of the lateral walls of the prosencephalic vesicle.
- contain **cerebral cortex, cerebral white matter, basal ganglia,** and **lateral ventricles**.
- are interconnected by three commissures: the corpus callosum, anterior commissure, and the hippocampal (fornical) commissure.
- Continuous hemispheric growth gives rise to **frontal, parietal, occipital,** and **temporal lobes,** which overlie the insula and dorsal brain stem.

B. Cerebral cortex (pallium)

- is formed by neuroblasts that migrate from the ventricular and intermediate layers to form a stratified subpial zone, the gray matter.
- is classified as neocortex and allocortex.

1. Neocortex (isocortex)

- is a six-layered cortex that represents 90% of the cortical mantle.

2. Allocortex

- is a three-layered cortex that represents 10% of the cortical mantle.
- is subdivided into the **archicortex,** which includes the hippocampal formation, and the **paleocortex,** which includes the olfactory cortex.

C. Corpus striatum (striatal eminence) [see Figure 7-8]

- appears in week 5 of development in the floor of the telencephalic vesicle.
- gives rise to the basal ganglia: the **caudate nucleus, putamen, amygdaloid nucleus,** and **claustrum**.
- is divided into the caudate nucleus and the lentiform nucleus by corticofugal and corticopetal fibers; these fibers make up the internal capsule.
- The neurons of the globus pallidus, a basal ganglion, have their origin in the subthalamus; they migrate into the telencephalic white matter and become the medial segments of the lentiform nucleus.

D. Commissures

- are fiber bundles that interconnect the hemispheres.
- cross the midline via the embryonic lamina terminalis (commissural plate).

1. Anterior commissure

- interconnects the olfactory structures and the middle and inferior temporal gyri.

2. Hippocampal (fornical) commissure

- interconnects the two hippocampi.

3. Corpus callosum

- appears between weeks 12 and 22 of development.
- is the largest commissure of the brain and interconnects homologous neocortical areas of the two cerebral hemispheres.
- does not project commissural fibers from the visual cortex (area 17) or the hand area of the motor or sensory strips (areas 4 and 3, 1, 2).

E. Gyri and fissures

- In month 4, no gyri or sulci are present; the brain is smooth, or lissencephalic.

– In month 8, all major sulci are present; the brain is convoluted, or gyrencephalic.

XII. Development of the Autonomic Nervous System

A. Sympathetic nervous system (Table 7-2)
– originates from the basal plate of the neural tube and neural crest cells

B. Parasympathetic nervous system (Table 7-3)
– originates from the basal plate of the neural tube and neural crest cells.

XIII. Development of the Cranial Nerves

A. Olfactory nerve (CN I)
– is derived from the **nasal (olfactory) placode**.
– mediates smell (olfaction).
– is capable of regeneration.

B. Optic nerve (CN II)
– is derived from the **ganglion cells of the retina**, a diverticulum of the diencephalon.
– mediates vision.
– does not regenerate after transection.

C. Oculomotor nerve (CN III)

– is derived from the **basal plate of the rostral midbrain**.

Table 7-2. Sympathetic Nervous System Embryonic Structures and Their Adult Derivatives

Embryonic Structure	Adult Derivative
Basal plate	Preganglionic sympathetic neurons within the intermediolateral cell column that form white communicating rami found between T1 and L3
Neural crest cells	Postganglionic sympathetic neurons within the sympathetic chain ganglia and prevertebral ganglia (e.g., celiac ganglia), chromaffin cells of adrenal medulla

Table 7-3. Parasympathetic Nervous System Embryonic Structures and Their Adult Derivatives

Embryonic Structure	Adult Derivative
Basal plate	Preganglionic parasympathetic neurons within the nuclei of the midbrain (CN III), pons (CN VII), and medulla (CN IX, X), and spinal cord at S2–S4
Neural crest cells	Postganglionic parasympathetic neurons within the ciliary (CN III), pterygopalatine (CN VII), submandibular (CN VII), otic (CN IX), enteric (CN X), and abdominal/pelvic cavity ganglia

– mediates ocular motility, pupillary constriction, and accommodation.

D. Trochlear nerve (CN IV)
– is derived from the **basal plate of the caudal midbrain**.
– innervates the superior oblique muscle.

E. Trigeminal nerve (CN V)
– Its motor division is derived from the **basal plate of the rostral pons**.
– Its sensory division is derived from the cranial neural crest.
– mediates the sensory and motor innervation of pharyngeal arch 1.

F. Abducent nerve (CN VI)
– is derived from the **basal plate of the caudal pons**.
– mediates abduction of the globe.

G. Facial nerve (CN VII)
– Its motor division is derived from the **basal plate of the pons**.
– Its sensory division is derived from the cranial **neural crest**.
– mediates the sensory and motor innervation of pharyngeal arch 2.

H. Vestibulocochlear nerve (CN VIII)
– is derived from the **otic placode**.
– Its vestibular division mediates balance and equilibrium.
– Its cochlear division mediates hearing.

I. Glossopharyngeal nerve (CN IX)
– Its motor division is derived from the **basal plate of the medulla**.
– Its sensory division is derived from the cranial **neural crest**.
– mediates the sensory and motor innervation of pharyngeal arch 3.

J. Vagal nerve (CN X)
– Its motor division is derived from the **basal plate of the medulla**.
– Its sensory division is derived from the cranial **neural crest**.
– mediates the sensory and motor innervation of pharyngeal arches 4 and 6.

K. Accessory nerve (CN XI)
– is derived from the **basal plate of the spinal segments C-1 to C-6**.
– innervates the sternocleidomastoid and trapezius muscles.

L. Hypoglossal nerve (CN XII)
– is derived from the **basal plate of the medulla**.
– innervates the intrinsic and extrinsic muscles of the tongue.

XIV. Development of the Choroid Plexus
– The choroid plexus develops from the **roof plates of the rhombencephalon and diencephalon**, and within the **choroid fissure of the telencephalon**.
– consists of modified ependymal cells and a vascular pia mater (tela choroidea), which invaginate into all ventricles.
– produces 500 ml of CSF per day. CSF is returned to the venous system via the arachnoid (granulations) villi of the venous dural sinuses (e.g., superior sagittal sinus).

XV. Congenital Malformations of the Central Nervous System

– result from failure of neural tube to close or separate from the surface ectoderm, or from failure of vertebral arches to fuse.

– Neural tube defects (e.g., spina bifida and anencephaly) may be diagnosed prenatally by detecting high alpha-fetoprotein levels in the amniotic fluid or in the maternal serum.

A. Spina bifida (Figure 7-10)

– usually occurs in the sacrolumbar region.

– includes the following variations:

1. Spina bifida occulta

– is a defect in the vertebral arches.

– is the least severe variation.

– occurs in 10% of the population.

2. Spina bifida with meningocele

– occurs when the meninges project through a vertebral defect, forming a sac filled with CSF.

– exists with the spinal cord remaining in its normal position.

3. Spina bifida with meningomyelocele

– occurs when the meninges and spinal cord project through a vertebral defect, forming a sac.

4. Spina bifida with myeloschisis

– is the most severe type of spina bifida.

– results in an **open neural tube** that lies on the surface of the back.

B. Ossification defects of the occipital bone (cranium bifidum) (Figure 7-11)

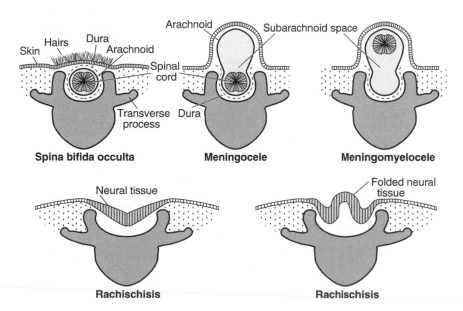

Figure 7-10. Schematic drawings illustrating the various types of spina bifida. (Modified from Sadler TW: *Langman's Medical Embryology*, 6th ed. Baltimore, Williams & Wilkins, 1990, p. 363.)

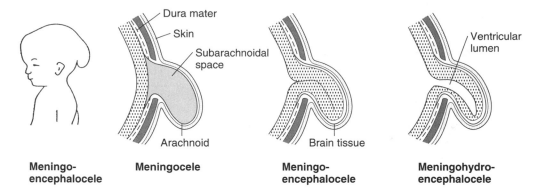

Figure 7-11. Schematic drawings illustrating the various types of occipital encephaloceles (cranium bifidum). (Adapted with permission from Sadler TW: *Langman's Medical Embryology*, 6th ed. Baltimore, Williams & Wilkins, 1990, p. 378.)

- occur once in every 2000 births.
- include the following variations: **cranial meningocele, meningoencephalocele,** and **meningohydroencephalocele.**

C. Anencephaly (meroanencephaly)

- results from failure of the anterior neuropore to close; the lamina terminalis fails to develop.
- occurs when the brain fails to develop; a rudimentary brain stem is usually present, and no cranial vault is formed.
- occurs once in every 1000 births.
- is the most common serious birth defect seen in stillborn fetuses.

D. Arnold-Chiari malformation (Figure 7-12)

- is a cerebellomedullary malformation, in which the caudal cerebellar vermis and tonsils and the medulla oblongata herniate through the foramen magnum.
- the outlet foramina of the fourth ventricle are obliterated, which results in an obstructive **hydrocephalus.**
- may cause stretching of the vagal and hypoglossal nerves, resulting in laryngeal stridor, spastic dysphonia, and respiratory embarrassment.
- is commonly associated with a lumbar **meningomyelocele** and **platybasia,** with malformation of the occipitovertebral joint; 50% have **aqueductal stenosis.**
- occurs once in every 1000 births.

E. Dandy-Walker syndrome (Figure 7-13)

- is a congenital hydrocephalus associated with **atresia of the outlet foramina of Luschka and Magendie.**
- is usually associated with dilatation of the fourth ventricle, agenesis of the cerebellar vermis, occipital meningocele, and frequently agenesis of the splenium of the corpus callosum.

F. Cystic malformations of the prosencephalon (Figure 7- 14)

1. Hydrocephalus

- is a dilation of the ventricles due to an excess of CSF.

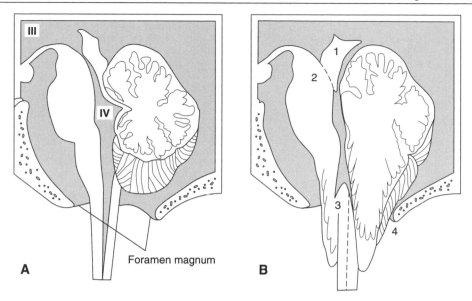

Figure 7-12. Arnold-Chiari malformation. Midsagittal section. *(A)* Normal cerebellum, fourth ventricle, and brain stem. *(B)* Abnormal cerebellum, fourth ventricle, and brain stem showing the common congenital anomalies: (1) beaking of the tectal plate; (2) aqueductal stenosis; (3) kinking and transforaminal herniation of the medulla into the vertebral canal; and (4) herniation of the cerebellar vermis and tonsils into the vertebral canal. An accompanying meningomyelocele is very common. (Reprinted with permission from Fix JD: *BRS Neuroanatomy.* Baltimore, Williams & Wilkins, 1996, p. 72.)

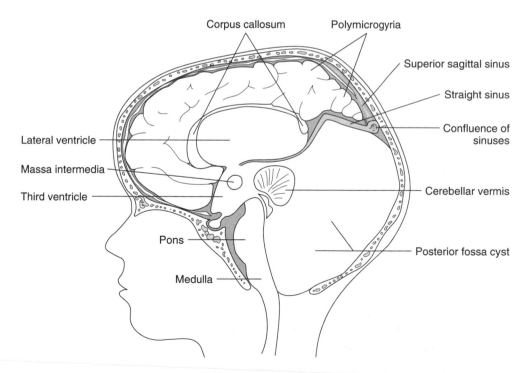

Figure 7-13. Dandy-Walker malformation. Midsagittal section. Consists of a large cyst in the posterior fossa, elevation of the confluence of the sinuses (torcular Herophili), agenesis or hypoplasia of the cerebellar vermis, hydrocephalus, and frequently agenesis or hypoplasia of the splenium of the corpus callosum. The Dandy-Walker malformation results from atresia of the outlet foramina of the fourth ventricle (Luschka and Magendie).

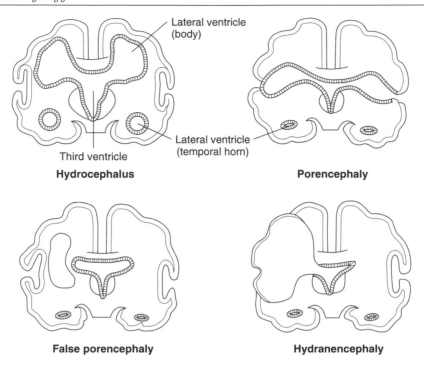

Figure 7-14. Cystic malformations of the prosencephalon (forebrain). Note the presence of the ependymal lining in these cysts. In hydranencephaly, the cyst is lined by glia and leptomeninges. In false porencephaly, the cyst is lined by glia.

- may result from blockage of CSF circulation (e.g., aqueductal stenosis) or overproduction of CSF (e.g., choroid plexus papilloma of lateral ventricle).
- **Aqueductal stenosis** is the most common cause of congenital hydrocephalus; it may be transmitted by an X-linked trait or may be caused by cytomegalovirus infection or toxoplasmosis.
- **Communicating hydrocephalus** results from obstruction distal to the ventricles.
- **Noncommunicating hydrocephalus** results from obstruction within the ventricle system (e.g., aqueductal occlusion).

2. Porencephaly

- bilateral porencephaly is called schizencephaly
- cystic cavitation of the cerebellum due to agenesis of the cordiale mantle
- the cavity is lined with ependyma and communicates with the lateral ventricle

3. False Porencephaly

- is a malformation consisting of cystic cavities that are lined with glia and do not communicate with the third ventricle

4. Hydranencephaly

- is the result of a destructive vascular lesion due to occlusion of the carotid arteries in utero
- widespread damage of the cortical mantle is seen in the territory of the carotid circulation

  – the vertebrobasilar system is spared; for example, the brain stem and the cerebellum
  – the fluid-filled cyst is covered by a glial layer; the cyst communicates with the lateral ventricle
  – other causes are toxoplasmosis, rubella, cytomegalovirus, and herpesvirus

G. Holoprosencephaly (arhinencephaly) (Figure 7-15)
  – results from failure of midline cleavage of the embryonic forebrain. The telencephalon contains a single ventricular cavity.
  – is characterized by the absence of olfactory bulbs and tracts (arhinencephaly).
  – is often seen in trisomy 13 (Patau syndrome).
  – may result from alcohol abuse during pregnancy, especially in the first 4 weeks of pregnancy.
  – is the most severe manifestation of **fetal alcohol syndrome**.

H. Megacolon (Hirschsprung's disease)
  – is also called congenital aganglionic megacolon (see Chapter 10).

I. Tethered spinal cord (filum terminale syndrome)
  – results from a thick and short filum terminale.
  – results in weakness and sensory deficits in the lower extremity and a neurogenic bladder.
  – is frequently associated with lipomatous tumors or lipomyelomeningoceles.
  – Deficits usually improve after transection.

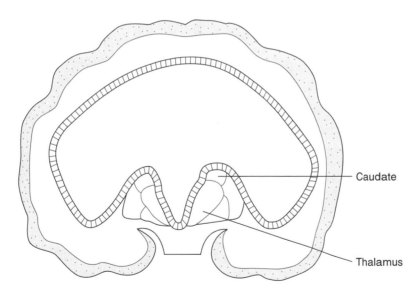

Figure 7-15. Holoprosencephaly results from failure of midline cleavage of the embryonic prosencephalon. The telencephalon contains a single ventricular cavity. It may result from alcohol abuse, especially during the first 4 weeks of pregnancy.

Review Test

Directions: Each of the numbered items or incomplete statements in this section is followed by answers or by completions of the statement. Select the **one** lettered answer or completion that is **best** in each case.

1. Which one of the following basal ganglia is NOT derived from the striatal eminence?

(A) Amygdaloid nucleus
(B) Head of the caudate nucleus
(C) Tail of the caudate nucleus
(D) Globus pallidus
(E) Putamen

2. When are the axons of the corticospinal tracts fully myelinated?

(A) In the late embryonic period
(B) In the mid-fetal period
(C) At birth
(D) By the end of the first postnatal year
(E) By the end of the second postnatal year

3. The medulla contains all of the following structures EXCEPT

(A) abducent nucleus
(B) nucleus ambiguus
(C) hypoglossal nucleus
(D) inferior olivary nucleus
(E) inferior salivatory nucleus

4. Alar plate derivatives of the metencephalon include all of the following structures EXCEPT

(A) the cerebellum
(B) the spinal trigeminal nucleus
(C) the principal trigeminal nucleus
(D) the superior salivatory nucleus
(E) the pontine nuclei

5. All of the following statements concerning the external granular layer of the cerebellum are correct EXCEPT

(A) it gives rise to granule cells
(B) it does not give rise to stellate cells
(C) it gives rise to Purkinje cells
(D) it is seen in the newborn
(E) it is thought to give rise to a medulloblastoma

6. Which of the following statements best describes the pathogenesis of hydranencephaly?

(A) Results from failure of midline cleavage of the embryonic forebrain
(B) Results from atresia of the outlet foramina of the fourth ventricle
(C) Results from blockage of the cerebral aqueduct
(D) Results from carotid artery occlusion
(E) Results from failure of the anterior neuropore to close

7. The anterior and posterior neuropores close during which week of embryonic development?

(A) Week 2
(B) Week 3
(C) Week 4
(D) Week 5
(E) Week 6

8. At birth the conus medullaris is found at which vertebral level?

(A) T-12
(B) L-1
(C) L-3
(D) S-1
(E) S-4

9. The telencephalon gives rise to all of the following EXCEPT

(A) the caudate nucleus
(B) the putamen
(C) the globus pallidus
(D) the claustrum
(E) the amygdala

10. Which of the following conditions results from failure of the anterior neuropore to close?

(A) Hydrocephalus
(B) Anencephaly
(C) Mongolism
(D) Craniosynostosis
(E) Meningoencephalocele

100

11. The diencephalon gives rise to all of the following structures EXCEPT

(A) mamillary bodies
(B) pineal body
(C) subthalamic nucleus
(D) adenohypophysis
(E) neurohypophysis

12. Caudal herniation of the cerebellar tonsils and medulla through the foramen magnum is called

(A) Dandy-Walker syndrome
(B) Down syndrome
(C) Arnold-Chiari syndrome
(D) cranium bifidum
(E) myeloschisis

13. The alar plate gives rise to all of the following EXCEPT

(A) the dentate nucleus
(B) the inferior olivary nucleus
(C) the gracile nucleus
(D) the nucleus ambiguus
(E) the cerebellar cortex

14. All of the following statements concerning myelination are correct EXCEPT

(A) it is accomplished by neural crest cells
(B) it is accomplished by Schwann cells in the peripheral nervous system (PNS)
(C) it is accomplished by oligodendrocytes in the central nervous system (CNS)
(D) it commences in the fourth fetal month
(E) it is completed by birth

15. All of the following statements concerning spina bifida are correct EXCEPT

(A) spina bifida results from failure of vertebral arches to fuse
(B) spina bifida is frequently associated with Arnold-Chiari malformation
(C) spina bifida usually occurs in the cervicothoracic region
(D) spina bifida occulta is the least severe variation
(E) spina bifida with myeloschisis is the most severe variation

16. The flexure that develops between the metencephalon and the myelencephalon is called the

(A) cephalic flexure
(B) mesencephalic flexure
(C) pontine flexure
(D) cerebellar flexure
(E) cervical flexure

17. All of the following statements concerning the neural tube are correct EXCEPT

(A) it lies between the surface ectoderm and the notochord
(B) it is completely closed by week 6 of development
(C) it contains the neural crest
(D) it gives rise to the central nervous system (CNS)
(E) it gives rise to myelin-producing cells

18. Which of the following statements best describes the sulcus limitans?

(A) It is found in the interpeduncular fossa
(B) It is located between the alar and basal plates
(C) It separates the medulla from the pons
(D) It separates the hypothalamus from the thalamus
(E) It separates the neocortex from the allocortex

19. The cerebellum develops from all of the following structures EXCEPT

(A) the rhombencephalon
(B) the metencephalon
(C) the rhombic lips
(D) the alar plates
(E) the myelencephalon

20. The neural crest gives rise to all of the following cells EXCEPT

(A) odontoblasts
(B) oligodendrocytes
(C) cells of enteric ganglia
(D) Schwann cells
(E) chromaffin cells

21. Myelinated preganglionic sympathetic neurons have their cell bodies in

(A) Clarke's column
(B) substantia gelatinosa
(C) intermediolateral cell column
(D) intermediomedial cell

22. Which one of the following ganglia does NOT give rise to postganglionic parasympathetic fibers?

(A) Celiac
(B) Ciliary
(C) Otic
(D) Pterygopalatine
(E) Submandibular

23. The choroid plexus of the fourth ventricle is derived from the

(A) alar plate
(B) basal plate
(C) floor plate
(D) rhombic lip
(E) roof plate

24. Tanycytes are found principally in the

(A) area postrema
(B) cerebral aqueduct
(C) lateral ventricles
(D) third ventricle
(E) fourth ventricle

Directions: Each group of items in this section consists of lettered options followed by a set of numbered items. For each item, select the **one** lettered option that is most closely associated with it. Each lettered option may be selected once, more than once, or not at all.

Questions 25–29

Match each description with the appropriate congenital malformation.

(A) Aqueductal stenosis
(B) Arnold-Chiari syndrome
(C) Dandy-Walker syndrome
(D) Hirschsprung's disease
(E) Meningohydroencephalocele

25. Herniation of brain tissue through a defect in occipital bone

26. Results from failure of neural crest cells to form the myenteric plexus

27. The most common cause of congenital hydrocephalus

28. Associated with atresia of the foramina of Luschka and Magendie

29. Frequently associated with platybasia and malformation of the occipitovertebral joint

Answers and Explanations

1–D. The globus pallidus has its origin in the subthalamus; neuroblasts from the subthalamus migrate into the telencephalic white matter to form the globus pallidus.

2–E. Axons of the corticospinal tracts are fully myelinated by the end of the second postnatal year; Babinski's sign (extensor plantar reflex) is usually not elicitable before myelination of the corticospinal tracts.

3–A. The abducent nucleus represents the general somatic efferent (GSE) column of the pons.

4–D. The superior salivatory nucleus represents the general visceral column of the pons. All somatic and visceral motor nuclei are derived from the basal plate. The cerebellum and pontine nuclei and the sensory nuclei of cranial nerves are derivatives of the alar plate.

5–C. New evidence documents that the external granular layer gives rise only to the granule cells of the internal granular layer and not to the basket (inner stellate) or stellate (outer stellate) neurons, as has long been thought.

6–D. Hydranencephaly consists of huge intracerebral cavitation resulting from infarction in the territory of the internal carotid artery; it may mimic ventricular dilation.

7–C. The anterior and posterior neuropores close during week 4 of development, the anterior on day 25, the posterior on day 27. Failure of the anterior neuropore to close results in anencephaly; failure of the posterior neuropore to close results in myeloschisis.

8–C. At birth, the conus medullaris extends to L-3, and in the adult it extends to the L1–L2 interspace. At 8 weeks, the spinal cord extends the entire length of the vertebral canal.

9–C. The globus pallidus develops from the diencephalon. Globus pallidus cells migrate from the subthalamus into the telencephalon.

10–B. Failure of the anterior neuropore to close results in anencephaly. The brain fails to develop; no cranial vault is formed.

11–D. The adenohypophysis (pars distalis, pars tuberalis, and pars intermedia) develops from Rathke's pouch, an ectodermal diverticulum of the stomodeum. The neurohypophysis develops from the infundibulum of the hypothalamus.

12–C. Arnold-Chiari syndrome is a cerebellomedullary malformation, in which the caudal vermis and medulla herniate through the foramen magnum, resulting in communicating hydrocephalus. Arnold-Chiari syndrome is frequently associated with spina bifida.

13–D. The alar plate of the mantle layer gives rise to sensory relay nuclei and the cerebellum. The nucleus ambiguus, a somatic visceral efferent (SVE) nucleus, is derived from the basal motor plate.

14–E. Myelination is not complete at birth. The corticospinal tracts are not completely myelinated until the end of the second postnatal year.

15–C. Spina bifida usually occurs in the sacrolumbar region.

16–C. The pontine flexure develops between the metencephalon (pons) and the myelencephalon (medulla). The pontine flexure results in lateral expansion of the walls of the metencephalon and myelencephalon, stretching of the roof of the fourth ventricle, and widening of the floor of the fourth ventricle (rhomboid fossa).

17–C. The neural tube, which lies between the surface ectoderm and the notochord, gives rise to the brain and spinal cord. Closure is already complete in week 5 of development. The neural crest lies between the neural tube and the surface ectoderm. The neural tube gives rise to oligodendrocytes, which produce the myelin of the central nervous system (CNS).

18–B. The sulcus limitans separates the sensory alar from the motor basal plates. It is found in the developing spinal cord and on the surface of the adult rhomboid fossa of the fourth ventricle. The bulbopontine sulcus (inferior pontine sulcus) separates the medulla from the pons. The hypothalamic sulcus separates the thalamus from the hypothalamus. The rhinal sulcus separates the neocortex from the allocortex.

19–E. The cerebellum arises from the alar plates of the rhombencephalon, which form the rhombic lips. The metencephalon, a division of the rhombencephalon, includes the pons and the cerebellum. The myelencephalon develops from the rhombencephalon and becomes the medulla oblongata.

20–B. The neural crest gives rise to dorsal root ganglion cells, the cells of the autonomic and enteric ganglia, Schwann cells, satellite cells, and chromaffin cells of the suprarenal medulla. The neural crest also gives rise to pigment cells (melanocytes), odontoblasts, meninges, and mesenchyme of the pharyngeal arches. Oligodendrocytes arise from glioblasts of the neural tube.

21–C. Myelinated preganglionic sympathetic neurons have their cell bodies in the intermediolateral cell column of the lateral horn; this cell column extends from C-8 to L-1. Myelinated preganglionic parasympathetic neurons have their cell bodies in the sacral autonomic nucleus, from S-2 to S-4.

22–A. The celiac ganglion is a preaortic (collateral) sympathetic ganglion; it gives rise to postganglionic sympathetic fibers.

23–E. The roof plate and its pial covering give rise to the choroid plexus, which invaginates into the fourth ventricle. The alar plate gives rise to sensory neurons; the basal plate gives rise to motor neurons; the floor plate contains decussating fibers; the rhombic lips give rise to the cerebellum.

24–D. Tanycytes are modified ependymal cells, found principally in the third ventricle. Tanycytes transport substances from the cerebrospinal fluid (CSF) to the hypophyseal portal system.

25–E. A meningohydroencephalocele consists of herniation of meninges, cerebellar tissue, and part of the fourth ventricle through an ossification defect in the occipital bone.

26–D. Hirschsprung's disease, congenital aganglionic megacolon, results from failure of neural crest cells to form the myenteric plexus of the sigmoid colon and rectum; patients present with fecal retention and abdominal distention.

27–A. The most common cause of congenital hydrocephalus is aqueductal stenosis; 50% of Arnold-Chiari malformations include aqueductal stenosis. Aqueductal stenosis may be transmitted by an X-linked trait, or it may be caused by cytomegalovirus infection or toxoplasmosis.

28–C. Dandy-Walker syndrome is congenital hydrocephalus associated with atresia of the outlet foramina of Luschka and Magendie; it is associated with agenesis of the cerebellar vermis and agenesis of the splenium of the corpus callosum.

29–B. Arnold-Chiari syndrome, a common congenital malformation, is frequently associated with platybasia and malformation of the occipitovertebral joint; other anomalies frequently seen are beaking of the tectum, aqueductal stenosis, kinking and herniation of the medulla, and herniation of the cerebellar vermis through the foramen magnum. Meningomyelocele (spina bifida) is a common component of the syndrome.

8

Ear

I. Overview
– The ear is the organ of **balance** and **hearing**.
– It consists of an **internal**, a **middle**, and an **external ear**. The gross anatomy of the ear is shown in Figure 8-1.

II. Internal Ear (Figures 8-1 and 8-2)
– develops in week 4 from a thickening of the **surface ectoderm** called the **otic placode**.
– The otic placode invaginates into the mesoderm adjacent to the rhombencephalon and becomes the **otic vesicle**.

A. Otic vesicle (see Figure 8-2)
– divides into **utricular** and **saccular portions**.

1. Utricular portion of the otic vesicle gives rise to:

a. Utricle

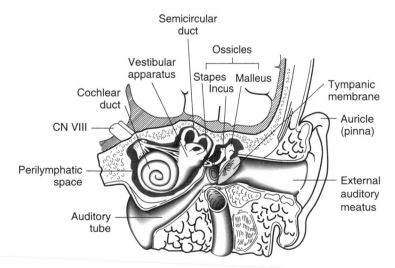

Figure 8-1. Gross anatomy of the ear, showing the three major divisions. (Reprinted from Johnson KE: *Human Developmental Anatomy.* Baltimore, Williams & Wilkins, 1988, p. 351.)

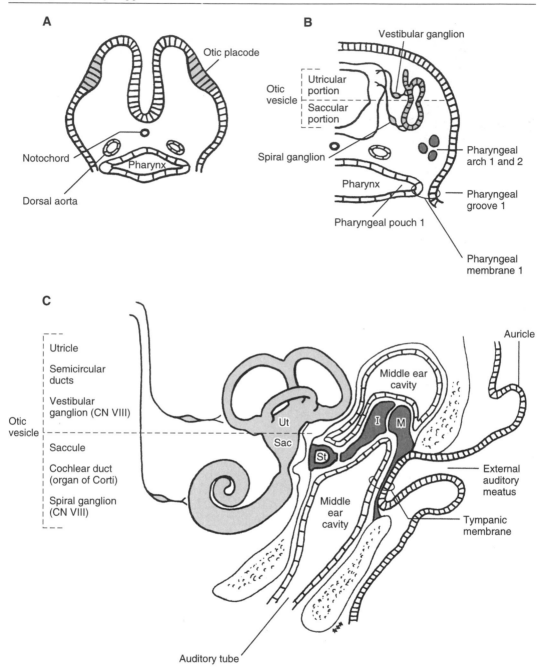

Figure 8-2. Schematic transverse sections showing the formation of the otic placode and otic vesicle from the surface ectoderm. *(A)* The otic placode invaginates into the mesoderm and becomes the otic vesicle. The mesoderm will later develop into bone, that is, the bony labyrinth. *(B)* The vestibular and spiral ganglia of CN VIII are derived from the otic vesicle. *(C)* The adult ear. *I* = incus; *M* = malleus; *Sac* = saccule; *St* = stapes; *Ut* = utricle. (Reprinted from Dudek RW: *High-Yield Embryology*. Baltimore, Williams & Wilkins, 1996, p. 45.)

- contains the sensory hair cells and otoliths of the macula utriculi.
- responds to linear acceleration and the force of gravity.

b. Semicircular ducts

- contain the sensory hair cells of the cristae ampullares.
- respond to angular acceleration.

c. Vestibular ganglion of CN VII, which lies at the base of the internal auditory meatus

d. Endolymphatic duct and sac

- is a membranous canal connecting with the saccule and utricle and terminating in a blind dilation beneath the dura.
- The endolymphatic sac absorbs endolymph.

2. **Saccular portion** of the otic vesicle gives rise to:

a. Saccule

- contains the sensory hair cells and otoliths of the macula sacculi.
- responds to linear acceleration and the force of gravity.

b. Cochlear duct (organ of Corti)

- has pitch (tonotopic) localization where high frequencies (20,000 Hz) are detected at the base and low frequencies (20 Hz) are detected at the apex.

c. Spiral ganglion of CN VII, which lies in the modiolus of the bony labyrinth.

B. The Membranous and Bony Labyrinth (see Figures 8-1 and 8-2)

1. The membranous labyrinth consists of all the structures derived from the otic vesicle (see Table 8-1).

Table 8-1. Embryonic Ear Structures and Their Adult Derivatives

Embryonic Structure	Adult Derivative
	Internal Ear
Otic vesicle	
Utricular portion	Utricle, semicircular ducts, vestibular ganglion of CN VIII, endolymphatic duct and sac
Saccular portion	Saccule, cochlear duct (organ of Corti) spiral ganglion of CN VIII
	Middle Ear
Pharyngeal arch 1	Malleus, incus, tensor tympani muscle
Pharyngeal arch 2	Stapes, stapedius muscle
Pharyngeal pouch 1	Auditory tube and middle ear cavity
Pharyngeal membrane 1	Tympanic membrane
	External Ear
Pharyngeal groove 1	External auditory meatus
Auricular hillocks	Auricle

CN = cranial nerve.

2. The membranous labyrinth is surrounded by mesoderm that becomes cartilaginous and then ossifies to become the **bony labyrinth** of the temporal bone.

3. The mesoderm closest to the membranous labyrinth degenerates, thus forming the **perilymphatic space** containing **perilymph**.

4. The membranous labyrinth is suspended within the bony labyrinth by perilymph.

5. Perilymph, which is similar in composition to cerebrospinal fluid (CSF), communicates with the subarachnoid space via the **perilymphatic duct**.

III. Middle Ear (see Figures 8-1 and 8-2)

A. Ossicles of the middle ear

1. Malleus

– develops from cartilage of **pharyngeal arch 1** (Meckel's cartilage).
– is attached to the tympanic membrane.
– is moved by the **tensor tympani muscle**, which is innervated by CN V-3.

2. Incus

– develops from the cartilage of **pharyngeal arch 1** (Meckel's cartilage).
– articulates with the malleus and stapes.

3. Stapes

– develops from the cartilage of **pharyngeal arch 2** (Reichert's cartilage).
– is moved by the **stapedius** muscle, which is innervated by CN VII.
– is attached to the oval window of the vestibule.

B. Auditory tube and middle ear cavity

– develops from **pharyngeal pouch 1**.

C. Tympanic membrane

– develops from **pharyngeal membrane 1**.
– separates the middle ear from the external auditory meatus of the external ear.
– is innervated by CN V-3 and CN IX.

IV. External Ear (see Figures 8-1 and 8-2)

A. External auditory meatus

– develops from the **pharyngeal groove 1**.
– becomes filled with ectodermal cells, forming a temporary **meatal plug** that disappears before birth.
– is innervated by **CN V-3** and **CN IX**.

B. Auricle

– develops from **six auricular hillocks** that surround pharyngeal groove 1.
– is innervated by **CN V-3, CN VII, CN IX, and CN X,** and **cervical nerves C-2 and C-3.**

V. Congenital Malformations of the Ear

A. Congenital deafness

– The organ of Corti may be damaged by exposure to **rubella virus**, especially during week 7 and week 8 of development.

B. Malformation of the auricles in chromosomal syndromes

– is seen in **Down syndrome** (trisomy 21), **Patau syndrome** (trisomy 13), and **Edwards syndrome** (trisomy 18).

C. Atresia of the external auditory meatus

– results from failure of the meatal plug to canalize; this is conduction deafness and is usually associated with the First Arch Syndrome.

D. Congenital cholesteatoma (epidermoid cyst)

– is a frequent cause of conduction deafness.
– is a benign tumor found in the tympanic cavity; is thought to develop from "epidermoid thickenings" of endodermal lining cells.

VI. Summary (Table 8-1)

Review Test

Directions: Each of the numbered items or incomplete statements in this section is negatively phrased, as indicated by an italicized word such as *not*, *least*, or *except*. Select the **one** lettered answer or completion that is **best** in each case.

1. All of the following statements concerning the cochlear duct are correct EXCEPT

(A) it arises from the otic vesicle
(B) it is of ectodermal origin
(C) it communicates with the saccule via the ductus reuniens
(D) it contains the spiral organ of Corti
(E) it contains perilymph

2. All of the following statements concerning the tympanic cavity are correct EXCEPT

(A) it is of mesodermal origin
(B) it develops from the tubotympanic recess
(C) the malleus and incus develop from pharyngeal arch 1
(D) the stapes develops from pharyngeal arch 2
(E) it communicates with the nasopharynx

3. All of the following statements concerning the otic vesicle are correct EXCEPT

(A) it gives rise to the membranous labyrinth
(B) it develops from the neuroectoderm
(C) it is found adjacent to the hindbrain
(D) it gives rise to the endolymphatic duct
(E) it gives rise to the cochlear duct

4. The auricle (pinna) of the external ear is innervated by all of the following nerves EXCEPT

(A) CN V-2
(B) CN V-3
(C) CN VII
(D) CN IX and X
(E) cervical nerves C-2 and C-3

5. All of the following statements concerning the auditory ossicles are correct EXCEPT

(A) the incus develops from Meckel's cartilage
(B) the malleus develops from the cartilage of pharyngeal arch 1
(C) the stapes is attached to the round window of the vestibule
(D) the muscle that moves the malleus is innervated by CN V-3
(E) the muscle that moves the stapes is innervated by CN VII

Directions: Each of the numbered items or incomplete statements in this section is followed by answers or by completions of the statement. Select the **one** lettered answer or completion that is **best** in each case.

6. The utricular portion of the otic vesicle gives rise to the

(A) ductus reuniens
(B) cochlear duct
(C) endolymphatic sac
(D) scala vestibuli
(E) scala tympani

7. The saccular portion of the otic vesicle gives rise to the

(A) organ of Corti
(B) endolymphatic duct
(C) superior semicircular canal
(D) crus commune nonampullare
(E) lateral semicircular canal

8. The tubotympanic recess gives rise to

(A) a conduit that interconnects the middle ear and the nasopharynx
(B) the external auditory meatus
(C) the internal auditory meatus
(D) the facial canal
(E) a conduit that interconnects the perilymphatic space with the subarachnoid space

9. Perilymph enters the subarachnoid space via the

(A) cochlear duct
(B) ductus reuniens
(C) perilymphatic duct
(D) vestibular aqueduct
(E) utriculosaccular duct

10. Pharyngeal groove 1 gives rise to the

(A) internal auditory meatus
(B) external auditory meatus
(C) eustachian tube
(D) cervical sinus
(E) primary tympanic cavity

Directions: The numbered items below correspond to lettered items in the figure. For each numbered item, select the **one** lettered option that is most closely associated with it. Each lettered option may be selected once, more than once, or not at all.

Questions 11–15

Match the following statements to the appropriate structure shown in the figure.

11. Is derived from pharyngeal arch 1

12. Contains the organ of Corti

13. Is derived from the pharyngeal pouch 1

14. Its sensory hair cells respond to linear acceleration

15. Contains otoliths

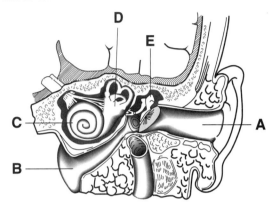

Reprinted from Johnson KE: *Human Developmental Anatomy.* Baltimore, Williams & Wilkins, 1988, p. 351.

Answers and Explanations

1–E. The cochlear duct is that part of the membranous labyrinth that contains the spiral organ of Corti. It contains endolymph, which is thought to be produced by the stria vascularis, the lateral wall of the cochlear duct.

2–A. The tympanic cavity develops from the tubotympanic recess; its epithelium is derived from the endoderm of pharyngeal pouch 1.

3–B. The otic vesicle arises from an invagination of the surface ectoderm, the otic placode.

4–A. The auricle (pinna) of the external ear is innervated by cranial nerves V-3 (mandibular division), VII, IX, and X; cervical nerves C-2 and C-3 also innervate the auricle.

5–C. The stapes is attached to the oval window of the vestibule.

6–C. The utricular region of the otic vesicle gives rise to the endolymphatic sac and duct, and semicircular ducts.

7–A. The saccular region of the otic vesicle gives rise to the cochlear duct, which houses the spiral organ of Corti.

8–A. The tubotympanic recess is derived from pharyngeal pouch 1. It gives rise to the tympanic cavity and the auditory (eustachian) tube; the auditory tube interconnects the tympanic cavity with the nasopharynx.

9–C. The perilymph enters the subarachnoid space of the posterior cranial fossa via the cochlear aqueduct, which contains the perilymphatic duct.

10–B. Pharyngeal groove 1 gives rise to the external auditory meatus.

11–E. The malleus is derived from the cartilage of pharyngeal arch 1.

12–C. The spiral organ of Corti is found in the cochlear duct.

13–B. The auditory (eustachian) tube is derived from pharyngeal pouch 1.

14–D. The sensory hair cells of the macula utriculi respond to linear acceleration and to the force of gravity.

15–D. The utricle contains a patch of sensory tissue called the macula utriculi; the macula contains sensory hair cells, a gelatinous layer, and otoliths (otoconia).

9

Eye

I. Development of the Optic Vesicle (Figure 9-1)

– begins at day 22 with the formation of **optic sulcus**, which evaginates from the wall of the diencephalon as the **optic vesicle** consisting of **neuroectoderm**.
– The optic vesicle invaginates and forms a double-layered **optic cup** and **optic stalk**.
– The double-layered optic cup consists of an **outer pigment layer** and **inner neural layer**.

A. Outer pigment layer of the optic cup

– gives rise to the pigment layer of the retina.

B. Intraretinal space

– separates the pigment layer of the retina from the neural layer of the retina.
– becomes a potential space.
– is a common site of retinal detachment.

C. Inner neural layer of the optic cup

– gives rise to the neural layer of the retina (i.e., the rods and cones, bipolar cells, and the ganglion cells).

D. Optic stalk

– contains the **choroid fissure** in which the **hyaloid vessels** are found that later become the **central artery and vein** of the retina.
– contains axons from the ganglion cell layer.
– the choroid fissure closes during week 7 so that the optic stalk, together with the axons of the ganglion cells, forms the **optic nerve (CN II), optic chiasm,** and **optic tract**.

E. Optic nerve (CN II)

– is a tract of the diencephalon.
– is not completely myelinated until 3 months after birth.
– is myelinated by oligodendrocytes.
– is not capable of regeneration after transection.
– is invested by the meninges and therefore is surrounded by a subarachnoid space (papilledema).

113

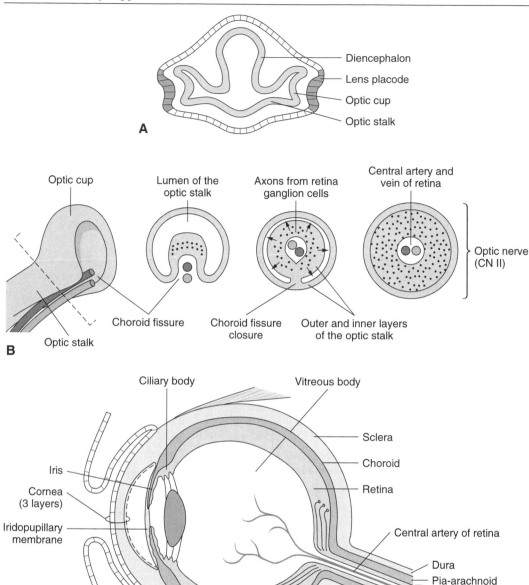

Figure 9-1. *(A)* The optic cup and optic stalk are evaginations of the diencephalon. The optic cup induces surface ectoderm to differentiate into the lens placode. *(B)* Formation of the optic nerve (CN II) from the optic stalk. The choroid fissure, which is located on the undersurface of the optic stalk, permits access of the hyaloid artery and vein to the inner aspect of the eye. The choroid fissue eventually closes. As ganglion cells form in the retina, axons accumulate in the optic stalk and cause the inner and outer layers of the optic stalk to fuse, obliterating the lumen and forming the optic nerve. *(C)* The adult eye. Note that the sclera is continuous with the dura mater and the choroid is continuous with the pia-arachnoid. The iridopupillary membrane is normally obliterated. (From Dudek RW: *High-Yield Embryology.* Baltimore, Williams & Wilkins, 1996, p 47.)

F. Iris (Figure 9-2)

  – The epithelium develops from the anterior portions of both the outer pigment layer and inner neural layer of the optic cup, which explains its histological appearance of two layers of columnar epithelium.
  – The stroma develops from mesoderm continuous with the choroid.
  – contains the **dilator pupillae muscle** and **sphincter pupillae muscle**, which are formed from the epithelium of the outer pigment layer by a transformation of these epithelial cells into contractile cells.

G. Ciliary body (see Figure 9-2)

  – The epithelium develops from the anterior portions of both the outer pigment layer and inner neural layer of the optic cup, which explains its histological appearance of two layers of columnar epithelium.
  – The stroma develops from mesoderm continuous with the choroid.
  – contains the **ciliary muscle**, which is formed from mesoderm within the choroid
  – contains **ciliary processes**.

  1. These produce **aqueous humor**, which circulates through the posterior and anterior chambers and drains into the venous circulation via the **trabecular meshwork** and the **canal of Schlemm**.

  2. They give rise to the **suspensory fibers** of the lens (ciliary zonule), which suspend the lens.

II. Development of Other Eye Structures

A. Sclera

  – develops from mesoderm surrounding the optic cup
  – forms an outer **fibrous** layer that is continuous with the dura mater posteriorly and the cornea anteriorly.

B. Choroid

  – develops from mesoderm surrounding the optic cup
  – forms an inner **vascular** layer that is continous with the pia-arachnoid posteriorly and iris/ciliary body anteriorly

C. Anterior chamber

  – develops from mesoderm over the anterior aspect of the eye that is continuous with the sclera and undergoes vacuolization to form a chamber.
  – The anterior chamber essentially splits the mesoderm into two layers:

  1. The mesoderm posterior to the anterior chamber is called the **iridopupillary membrane**, which is normally resorbed prior to birth.

  2. The mesoderm anterior to the anterior chamber develops into the **substantia propria of the cornea** and **corneal endothelium**.

D. Cornea

  – develops from both surface ectoderm and mesoderm lying anterior to the anterior chamber.
  – The surface ectoderm forms the **anterior epithelium of the cornea**.

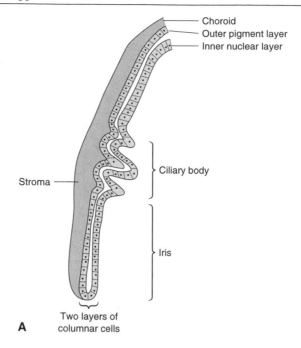

Choroid
Outer pigment layer
Inner nuclear layer

Ciliary body

Stroma

Iris

Two layers of
columnar cells

A

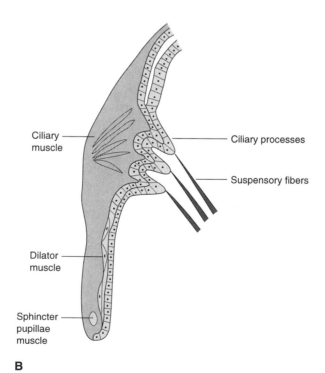

Ciliary
muscle

Ciliary processes

Suspensory fibers

Dilator
muscle

Sphincter
pupillae
muscle

B

Figure 9-2. (*A* and *B*) Sagittal sections through the developing iris and ciliary body. The iris and ciliary body form from the outer pigment layer and inner neural layer of the optic cup. In the adult, this embryological origin is reflected histologically by two layers of columnar epithelium that line both the iris and ciliary body.

– The mesoderm forms the **substantia propria of the cornea** and **corneal endothelium**.

E. Lens

– develops from surface ectoderm which forms the **lens placode**.
– The lens placode invaginates to form the **lens vesicle**.
– The cells of the posterior wall of the lens vesicle elongate, lose their nuclei, and form the lens fibers of the adult lens.

F. Vitreous body

– develops from mesoderm that migrates through the choroid fissure and forms a transparent gelatinous substance between the lens and retina.
– contains the **hyaloid artery**, which later obliterates to form the **hyaloid canal** of the adult eye.

G. Canal of Schlemm

– is found at the sclerocorneal junction called the limbus.
– drains the aqueous humor into the venous circulation.
– obstruction results in increased intraocular pressure (**glaucoma**).

H. Extraocular muscles

– develop from mesoderm surrounding the optic cup that has been called "preotic myotomes (somites)," although in man the origin is still controversial.

III. Congenital Malformations of the Eye

A. Coloboma iridis (Figure 9-3A)

– is a cleft in the iris caused by failure of the choroid fissure to close in week 7 of development.
– may extend into the ciliary body, retina, choroid, or optic nerve.
– Palpebral coloboma, a notch in the eyelid, results from a defect in the developing eyelid.

B. Persistent iridopupillary membrane (Figure 9-3B)

– consists of strands of connective tissue that partially cover the pupil; seldom affects vision.

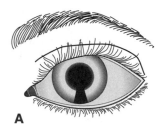 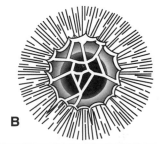

Figure 9-3. *(A)* Coloboma iridis; results from failure of the choroid fissure to close. *(B)* Partially persistent iridopupillary membrane; normally, this membrane is totally resorbed at birth.

C. Congenital cataracts

– are opacities of the lens, usually bilateral.

– are common and may result from the following:

1. Rubella virus infection, toxoplasmosis, or congenital syphilis

2. Down syndrome (trisomy 21)

3. Galactosemia, an inborn error of metabolism

D. Congenital glaucoma (buphthalmos)

– is increased intraocular pressure due to abnormal development of the canal of Schlemm or the iridocorneal filtration angle.

– is usually genetically determined.

– may result from maternal rubella infection.

E. Microphthalmia

– is a small eye, usually associated with intrauterine infections from the TORCH group of microorganisms (*Toxoplasma*, rubella virus, cytomegalovirus, and herpes simplex virus).

F. Anophthalmia

– is absence of the eye.

– is due to failure of the optic vesicle to form.

G. Cyclopia

– is a single orbit and one eye.

– is due to failure of median cerebral structures to develop.

H. Retinocele

– results from herniation of the retina into the sclera.

– results from failure of the choroid fissure to close.

I. Retrolental fibroplasia (retinopathy of prematurity)

– is an oxygen-induced retinopathy seen in premature infants.

J. Detached retina

– may result from head trauma or may be congenital.

– The site of detachment is between the outer and inner layers of the optic cup (i.e., between the retinal pigment epithelial layer and outer segment layer of rods and cones of the neural retina).

K. Papilledema

– is edema of the optic disk (papilla) due to increased intracranial pressure; this pressure is reflected into the subarachnoid space, which surrounds the optic nerve (CN II).

L. Retinitis pigmentosa

– is hereditary degeneration and atrophy of the retina.

– may be transmitted as an autosomal recessive, autosomal dominant, or X-linked trait.

– is characterized by a degeneration of the rods, night blindness (nyctalopia), and "gun barrel vision."

– may be due to abetalipoproteinemia (Bassen-Kornzweig syndrome); progression of this disease may be arrested with massive doses of vitamin A.

IV. Summary (Table 9-1)

Table 9-1. Embryonic Eye Structures and Their Adult Derivatives

Embryonic Structure	Adult Derivative
Diencephalon (neuroectoderm) Optic cup	Retina, iris epithelium, dilator and sphincter pupillae muscles, ciliary body epithelium
Optic stalk	Optic nerve (CN II), optic chiasm, optic tract
Surface ectoderm	Lens, anterior epithelium of cornea
Mesoderm	Sclera, choroid, stroma of iris, stroma of ciliary body, ciliary muscle, substantia propria of cornea, corneal endothelium, vitreous body, central artery and vein of retina, extraocular muscles

Review Test

Directions: Each of the numbered items or incomplete statements in this section is followed by answers or by completions of the statement. Select the **one** lettered answer or completion that is **best** in each case.

1. The surface ectoderm gives rise to the

(A) dilator pupillae muscle
(B) retina
(C) lens
(D) sclera
(E) choroid

2. Failure of the choroid fissure to close results in

(A) congenital detached retina
(B) congenital aniridia
(C) congenital aphakia
(D) coloboma iridis
(E) microphthalmos

3. All of the following statements concerning the optic cup are correct EXCEPT

(A) develops from the optic vesicle
(B) is a telencephalic structure
(C) gives rise to the pigment layer of the retina
(D) gives rise to the neural layer of the retina
(E) gives rise to the sphincter pupillae muscle

4. All of the following statements concerning the ciliary body are correct EXCEPT

(A) is derived from two sources
(B) plays a role in accommodation
(C) produces aqueous humor
(D) gives rise to the suspensory ligament
(E) contains the hyaloid canal

5. Hyperoxygenation of premature infants may result in

(A) congenital glaucoma
(B) microphthalmia
(C) coloboma
(D) retrolental fibroplasia
(E) persistent pupillary membrane

6. All of the following statements concerning the optic nerve are correct EXCEPT

(A) develops from the optic stalk
(B) is not a true peripheral nerve
(C) its axons are fully myelinated at birth
(D) is surrounded by the meninges
(E) normally there are no myelinated axons found within the retina

7. The hyaloid canal is found in the

(A) vitreous body
(B) choroid
(C) optic stalk
(D) ciliary body
(E) intraretinal space

8. Aqueous humor is produced by the

(A) choroid plexus
(B) trabecular meshwork
(C) ciliary processes
(D) vitreous body
(E) lens vesicle

9. Aqueous humor enters the venous circulation via

(A) arachnoid villi
(B) scleral canal
(C) hyaloid canal
(D) canal of Schlemm
(E) Cloquet's canal

10. In a detached retina, the site of detachment is found

(A) within the outer plexiform layer
(B) within the inner plexiform layer
(C) between the inner nuclear layer and the outer nuclear layer
(D) between the choriocapillaris and the pigment epithelial layer
(E) between the pigment epithelial layer and the layer of outer segments of rods and cones

Directions: The numbered items below correspond to lettered items in the figure. For each numbered item, select the **one** lettered option that is most closely associated with it. Each lettered option may be selected once, more than once, or not at all.

Questions 11–16

Match the following statements with the appropriate embryological structures shown in the figure.

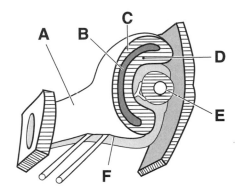

Modified from Moore KL and Persaud TVN: *The Developing Human,* 5th ed. Philadelphia, WB Saunders, 1993, p 436.

11. Is derived from the surface ectoderm

12. Becomes the second cranial nerve (CN II)

13. Gives rise to the pigment epithelium of the retina

14. Failure of this structure to fuse results in coloboma iridis

15. Detachment of the retina occurs at this site

16. Contains the rods and cones

Answers and Explanations

1–C. The lens forms from the lens placode that is induced by the optic cup.

2–D. Failure of the choroid (optic) fissure to close results in a cleft of the iris, a coloboma iridis. This defect may extend into the ciliary body, choroid, optic nerve, or retina. Congenital aphakia, absence of the lens, may result from defective development of the lens placode.

3–B. The optic cup and its derivatives, the retina and optic nerve, develop from the diencephalon.

4–E. The hyaloid canal is a rudiment of the obliterated hyaloid vessels found in the vitreous body. The ciliary body is derived from the anterior two layers of the optic cup (neuroectoderm) and from an anterior extension of the choroid (mesoderm).

5–D. Retrolental fibroplasia results from hyperoxygenation of premature infants. In premature infants, high oxygen concentration results in vaso-obliteration of the terminal arterioles, leading to hemorrhage and infarction of the retina. This phenomenon is peculiar to the incompletely vascularized peripheral retina.

6–C. The axons of the optic nerve are not completely myelinated until 3 months after birth. Myelinated axons are normally not found in the retina. The optic nerve is not a true peripheral nerve but a tract of the diencephalon; when severed, the optic nerve does not regenerate. Myelination in the central nervous system (CNS) is accomplished by oligodendrocytes; oligodendrocytes are not found in the retina.

7–A. The hyaloid canal (Cloquet's canal) is found in the vitreous body. In early development, a hyaloid artery passes through the vitreous body to perfuse the developing lens; in the late fetal period, this artery obliterates to form the hyaloid canal.

8–C. Aqueous humor is produced by the ciliary processes of the ciliary body. It flows from the posterior chamber, through the pupil, into the anterior chamber and finally to the canal of Schlemm, which empties into the extraocular veins.

9–D. Aqueous humor enters the venous circulation via the canal of Schlemm. Blockage of this canal results in increased intraocular pressure (glaucoma).

10–E. The site of retinal detachment is between the pigment epithelial layer and the layer of outer segments of rods and cones; this corresponds to the intraretinal space between the inner and outer layers of the optic cup. Retinal detachment occurs when fluid from the vitreous compartment passes through a retinal hole and separates the pigment epithelial layer from the layer of outer segments of rods and cones.

11–E. The lens vesicle is derived from the surface ectoderm.

12–A. The optic stalk becomes the second cranial nerve (CN II). The optic nerve is a tract of the central nervous system (CNS) that terminates in the thalamus (lateral geniculate body).

13–C. The outer layer of the optic cup gives rise to the pigment epithelium of the retina.

14–F. Failure of the optic (choroid) fissure to close during week 7 of development results in a coloboma of the iris; this cleft may extend into the ciliary body, retina, and choroid. The optic fissure contains the hyaloid vessels, which become the central artery and vein of the retina.

15–B. Detachment of the retina occurs between the pigment epithelium layer and the layer of outer segments of rods and cones. In the embryo the pigment layer is separated from the neural layer by the intraretinal space.

16–D. The inner layer of the optic cup gives rise to the neural layer of the retina and includes the rods and cones, the bipolar cells, and the ganglion cells.

10

Digestive System

I. Overview

A. Development of the primitive gut tube (Figure 10-1)

– The gut tube is formed from the incorporation of the dorsal part of the yolk sac into the embryo due to the craniocaudal folding and lateral folding of the embryo.

– The **primitive gut tube** extends from the oropharyngeal membrane to the cloacal membrane and is divided into the **foregut, midgut,** and **hindgut**.

– The derivatives of the primitive gut tube are summarized in Table 10-1.

B. Adult histology of gastrointestinal tract versus embryology (Figure 10-2)

1. Histologically, the general plan of the adult gastrointestinal tract consists of a **mucosa** (epithelial lining and glands, lamina propria, and muscularis mucosae), **submucosa, muscularis externa**, and **adventitia** or **serosa**.

2. Embryologically, the epithelial lining and glands of the mucosa are derived from endoderm, whereas the other components are derived from visceral mesoderm.

II. Derivatives of the Foregut

– These are supplied by the **celiac trunk**. (*Note:* The exception to this is the esophagus; the intra-abdominal portion of the esophagus is supplied by the celiac trunk, but the intrathoracic portion is supplied by other branches of the aorta.)

– The terminal end of the foregut contacts the surface ectoderm of the stomodeum to form the oropharyngeal membrane.

A. Esophagus

1. Development

– The foregut is divided into the **esophagus** dorsally and the **trachea** ventrally by the **tracheoesophageal folds**, which fuse to form the **tracheoesophageal septum**.

– The esophagus is initially short but lengthens with descent of the heart and lungs.

123

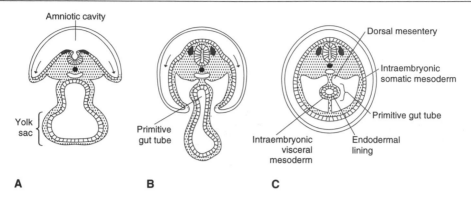

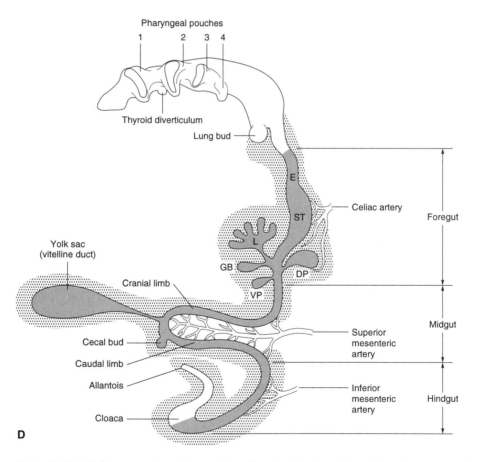

Figure 10-1. *(A, B, C)* Cross sections of an embryo showing the formation of the primitive gut tube. *(D)* Longitudinal view of the entire primitive gut tube. *Arrowed lines* indicate the foregut, midgut, and hindgut divisions. *Shaded area* indicates that portion of the gut tube that is involved in formation of the digestive system. *Stippled area* indicates visceral mesoderm. *White areas* indicate portions of the primitive gut tube involved in the formation of the thyroid gland, pharyngeal pouches, lungs, and urogenital system. *DP* = dorsal pancreatic bud; *E* = esophagus; *GB* = gallbladder; *L* = liver; *ST* = stomach; *VP* = ventral pancreatic bud.

Table 10-1. Derivatives of the Primitive Gut Tube

Foregut	Midgut	Hindgut
Thyroid*		
Pharyngeal pouches*	Lower duodenum	Distal one-third of transverse colon
Lungs †	Jejunum	
Esophagus	Ileum	Descending colon
Stomach	Cecum	Sigmoid colon
Liver	Appendix	Rectum
Gallbladder and bile ducts	Ascending colon	Upper part of anal canal
Pancreas	Proximal two-thirds of transverse colon	Urogenital derivatives ‡
Upper duodenum		

* See Chapter 12.
† See Chapter 11.
‡ See Chapters 13, 14, and 15.

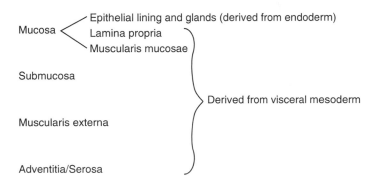

Figure 10-2. Diagram showing the general plan of histologic and embryologic organization of the adult gastrointestinal tract.

– During development, the endodermal lining of the esophagus proliferates rapidly and obliterates the lumen; later **recanalization** occurs.

2. **Sources**

– **Stratified squamous epithelium, mucosal glands,** and **submucosal glands** of the definitive esophagus are derived from endoderm.

– Lamina propria, muscularis mucosa, submucosa, skeletal muscle (upper one-third) and smooth muscle (lower two-thirds) of muscularis externa, and adventitia of the definitive esophagus are derived from visceral mesoderm.

3. **Clinical considerations**

a. **Esophageal atresia**

– occurs when the tracheoesophageal septum deviates too far dorsally, causing the esophagus to end as a closed tube.

– is associated clinically with **polyhydramnios** (fetus is unable to swallow amniotic fluid) and **tracheoesophageal fistula**.

b. **Esophageal stenosis**

– occurs when the lumen of the esophagus is narrowed as a result of incomplete recanalization.

B. Stomach (Figure 10-3)

1. Development

a. A fusiform dilatation forms in the foregut in week 4; this gives rise to the primitive stomach.

b. The dorsal part of the primitive stomach grows faster than the ventral part, thereby resulting in the greater and lesser curvatures, respectively.

c. The primitive stomach rotates 90° clockwise around its longitudinal axis.

– The 90° rotation affects all foregut structures and is responsible for the adult anatomic relationship of foregut viscera.

– As a result of this clockwise rotation:

(1) **The dorsal mesentery** is carried to the left and eventually forms the **greater omentum**.

(2) **The left vagus nerve** innervates the ventral surface of the stomach, and the **right vagus nerve** innervates the dorsal surface.

2. Sources

– **Surface mucous cells** lining the stomach, **mucous neck cells, parietal cells, chief cells,** and **enteroendocrine cells** comprising the gastric glands of the definitive stomach are derived from endoderm.

– The lamina propria; muscularis mucosae; submucosa; the outer longitudinal, middle circular, and inner oblique layers of smooth muscle of the muscularis externa; and the serosa of the definitive stomach are derived from visceral mesoderm.

3. Clinical considerations: Hypertrophic pyloric stenosis

– occurs when the muscle layer in the pyloric region hypertrophies, causing a narrow pyloric lumen that obstructs food passage.

– is associated clinically with **projectile vomiting after feeding** and **palpation of a small knot at the right costal margin**.

– Other stomach malformations are rare.

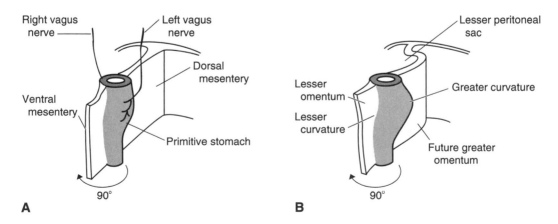

Figure 10-3. Diagram depicting the development and 90° rotation of the stomach at week 4 *(A)* and at week 6 *(B)*.

C. Liver (Figure 10-4)

1. Development

  a. The endodermal lining of the foregut forms an outgrowth into the surrounding mesoderm called the **hepatic diverticulum**. (*Note:* The mesoderm in the vicinity of the developing liver is actually the **septum transversum**, which is involved in the formation of the diaphragm. This explains the intimate gross anatomic relationship between the liver and diaphragm.)

  b. Cords of cells (**hepatic cords**) from the hepatic diverticulum grow into the surrounding **septum transversum**.

  c. Hepatic cords arrange themselves around the **vitelline and umbilical veins**, which course through the septum transversum and form the **hepatic sinusoids**.

  d. Due to the tremendous growth of the liver, it bulges into the abdominal cavity, thereby stretching the septum transversum to form the **ventral mesentery**, consisting of the **falciform ligament** and the **lesser omentum**.

  – The lesser omentum can be divided into the **hepatogastric ligament** and **hepatoduodenal ligament**.

  – The falciform ligament contains the left umbilical vein; the lesser omentum contains the bile duct, portal vein, and hepatic artery.

2. Sources

  – **Hepatocytes** and the **simple columnar** or **cuboidal epithelium** lining the biliary tree of the definitive liver are derived from endoderm.

  – **Kupffer cells, hematopoietic cells, endothelium of the sinusoids,** and **fibroblasts (connective tissue)** of the definitive liver are derived from mesoderm.

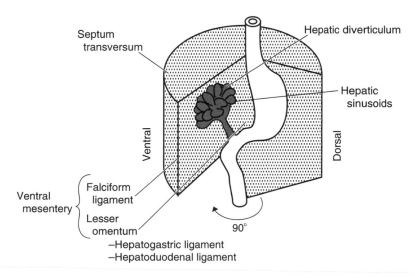

Figure 10-4. Diagram depicting the formation of the liver. *Shaded area* indicates the hepatic diverticulum, and *stippled area* indicates surrounding mesoderm. The liver area is the only area where the ventral mesentery persists.

3. Clinical considerations

– Congenital malformations of the liver are rare except for minor gross anatomic variations.

D. Gallbladder and extrahepatic bile ducts (Figure 10-5)

1. Development

– The connection between the hepatic diverticulum and the foregut narrows to form the **bile duct**.

– An outgrowth from the bile duct gives rise to the **gallbladder** and **cystic duct**.

– The cystic duct divides the bile duct into the **hepatic duct** and **common bile duct**.

– During development, the endodermal lining of the gallbladder and extrahepatic bile ducts proliferates rapidly and obliterates the lumen; later **recanalization** occurs.

2. Sources

– **Simple columnar epithelium** and **mucosal glands** lining the definitive gallbladder and **simple columnar or cuboidal epithelium** lining the definitive extrahepatic bile ducts are derived from endoderm.

– Lamina propria, muscularis externa, and adventitia of the definitive gallbladder are derived from visceral mesoderm. (*Note:* There is no muscularis mucosae or submucosa in the gallbladder.)

3. Clinical considerations

a. Extrahepatic biliary atresia

– occurs when the lumen of the ducts is obliterated as a result of incomplete recanalization.

– is associated clinically with **jaundice soon after birth**, **white clay-colored stool**, and **dark-colored urine**.

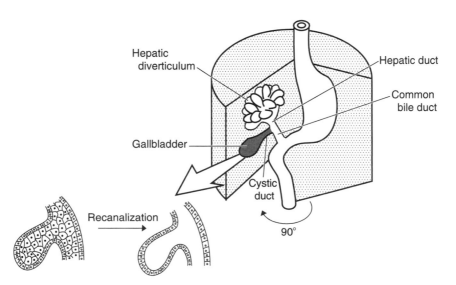

Figure 10-5. Diagram depicting the development of the gallbladder and extrahepatic bile ducts *(shaded area)*. *Large arrow* indicates the recanalization process. *Stippled area* indicates surrounding mesoderm.

  b. Other gallbladder malformations are rare except for minor gross anatomic variations.

E. Pancreas (Figure 10-6)

  1. Development

  a. The endodermal lining of the foregut forms two outgrowths, the **ventral pancreatic bud** and the **dorsal pancreatic bud**.

  b. Within both pancreatic buds, endodermal tubules surrounded by mesoderm branch repeatedly to form **acinar cells and ducts (exocrine pancreas)**; isolated clumps of cells bud from the tubules and accumulate within the mesoderm to form **islet cells (endocrine pancreas)**.

  c. Because of the 90° clockwise rotation of the duodenum, the ventral bud rotates dorsally and fuses with the dorsal bud to form the definitive adult pancreas.

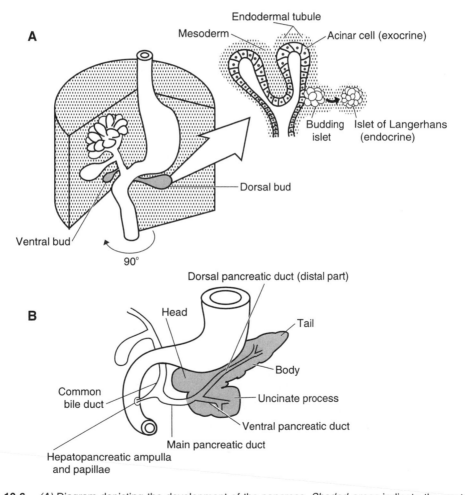

Figure 10-6. *(A)* Diagram depicting the development of the pancreas. *Shaded areas* indicate the ventral and dorsal pancreatic buds. *Stippled area* indicates surrounding mesoderm. Enlargement shows formation of pancreatic islets. *(B)* Diagram showing the adult anatomic relationships of this area. Note the common bile duct passing dorsal to the duodenum due to the 90° rotation.

(1) The ventral bud forms the **uncinate process** and **a portion of the head of the pancreas**.

(2) The dorsal bud forms the **remaining portion of the head, body,** and **tail of the pancreas**.

(3) The **main pancreatic duct** is formed from the distal part of the dorsal pancreatic duct and the entire ventral pancreatic duct.

(4) The main pancreatic duct and common bile duct form a single opening (**hepatopancreatic ampulla of Vater**) into the duodenum at the tip of a large papillae (**hepatopancreatic papillae**).

2. Sources

– **Acinar cells, islet cells**, and **simple columnar or cuboidal epithelium** lining the pancreatic ducts of the definitive pancreas are derived from endoderm.

– Surrounding connective tissue and vascular components of the definitive pancreas are derived from visceral mesoderm.

3. Clinical considerations

a. Annular pancreas

– occurs when the ventral pancreatic bud fuses with the dorsal bud both dorsally and ventrally, thereby forming a ring of pancreatic tissue around the duodenum.

– is associated clinically with **obstruction of the duodenum** shortly after birth.

b. Accessory pancreatic duct

– develops when the proximal part of the dorsal bud duct persists and enters the duodenum at its own site.

c. Accelerated development of pancreatic islets

– occurs when fetal islets are exposed to high blood glucose levels, such as those present in a pregnancy involving a diabetic woman.

– Glucose freely crosses the placenta and stimulates fetal insulin secretion, which causes increased fat and glycogen deposition in fetal tissues.

– is associated clinically with **increased birth weight of infant at term**.

F. Upper duodenum

– develops from the caudalmost part of the foregut.

III. Derivatives of the Midgut

– These are supplied by the **superior mesenteric artery**.

A. Lower duodenum

1. Development

– develops from the most cranial part of the midgut.

– The junction of the upper and lower duodenum is just distal to the opening of the common bile duct.

– During development, the endodermal lining of the duodenum proliferates rapidly and obliterates the lumen; later recanalization occurs.

2. Clinical considerations

a. Duodenal stenosis

– occurs when the lumen of the duodenum is narrowed as a result of incomplete recanalization.

b. Duodenal atresia

– occurs when the lumen of the duodenum is occluded as a result of failed recanalization.

– is associated clinically with **polyhydramnios, bile-containing vomitus**, and a **distended stomach**.

B. Jejunum, ileum, cecum, appendix, ascending colon, and the proximal two-thirds of the transverse colon (Figure 10-7)

1. Development

a. The midgut forms a U-shaped loop (**midgut loop**) that herniates through the primitive umbilical ring into the extraembryonic coelom (**physiologic umbilical herniation**) beginning at week 6.

b. The midgut loop consists of a **cranial limb** and a **caudal limb**.

(1) The cranial limb forms the **jejunum** and **upper part of the ileum**.

(2) The caudal limb forms the **cecal diverticulum**, from which the **cecum** and **appendix** develop; the rest of the caudal limb forms the **lower part of the ileum, ascending colon,** and **proximal two-thirds of the transverse colon**.

c. The midgut loop rotates a total of **270° counterclockwise** around the superior mesenteric artery as it returns to the abdominal cavity, thus reducing the physiologic herniation, around week 11.

2. Sources

– **Simple columnar absorptive cells** lining midgut derivatives, **goblet cells, Paneth cells**, and **enteroendocrine cells** comprising the intestinal glands are derived from endoderm.

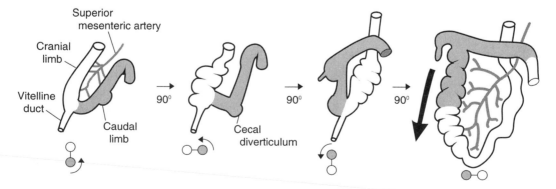

Figure 10-7. Diagram depicting the 270° counterclockwise rotation of the midgut loop. Shaded area indicates the caudal limb. Note that after the 270° rotation, the cecum and appendix are located in the upper abdominal cavity. Later in development, there is growth in the direction indicated by the *bold arrow* so that the cecum and appendix end up in the lower abdominal cavity.

– Lamina propria, muscularis mucosae, submucosa, inner circular and outer longitudinal smooth muscle of the muscularis externa, and serosa are derived from visceral mesoderm.

3. Clinical considerations

a. Omphalocele
– occurs when the intestines (midgut loop) fail to return to the abdominal cavity.
– presents in the newborn as a **light gray, shiny sac** protruding from the base of the umbilical cord.

b. Ileal diverticulum (Meckel's diverticulum)
– occurs when a remnant of the vitelline duct persists, thereby forming an outpouching from the ileum.
– The outpouching may connect to the umbilicus via a fibrous cord or fistula.
– is associated clinically with symptoms resembling **appendicitis**.

c. Vitelline fistula
– occurs when the vitelline duct remains open, thereby forming a direct communication between the lumen of the ileum and the exterior of the body at the umbilicus.
– A **fecal discharge** at the umbilicus may be observed.

d. Gastroschisis
– occurs when there is a defect in the ventral abdominal wall, allowing **protrusion of the viscera**.

e. Nonrotation of the midgut
– occurs when the midgut rotates only 90° counterclockwise, thereby positioning the small intestine entirely on the right side and the large intestine entirely on the left side.

f. Malrotation of the midgut
– occurs when the midgut undergoes partial counterclockwise rotation, resulting in the cecum and appendix lying in the upper part of the abdominal cavity.
– is associated clinically with **volvulus** (twisting of the intestines), which obstructs passage of intestinal contents and may cause necrosis due to compromised blood supply. (*Note:* The abnormal position of the appendix due to malrotation of the midgut should be considered when diagnosing appendicitis.)

g. Intestinal stenosis
– occurs when the lumen of the intestines is narrowed as a result of incomplete recanalization.

h. Intestinal atresia
– occurs when the lumen of the intestines is occluded as a result of failed recanalization.

i. Duplication of the intestines
– occurs when a segment of the intestines is duplicated as a result of abnormal recanalization.

j. Retrocecal and retrocolic appendix

– occurs when the appendix is located on the **posterior side** of the cecum or colon. (*Note:* The appendix is normally found on the **medial side** of the cecum. However, this misplacement is very common and is important to remember during appendectomies.)

IV. Derivatives of the Hindgut (Figure 10-8)

– These are supplied by the **inferior mesenteric artery**.
– include the **distal one-third of the transverse colon, descending colon, sigmoid colon, rectum,** and **upper anal canal.**

A. Development

1. The cranial end of the hindgut develops into the **distal one-third of the transverse colon, descending colon,** and **sigmoid colon.**

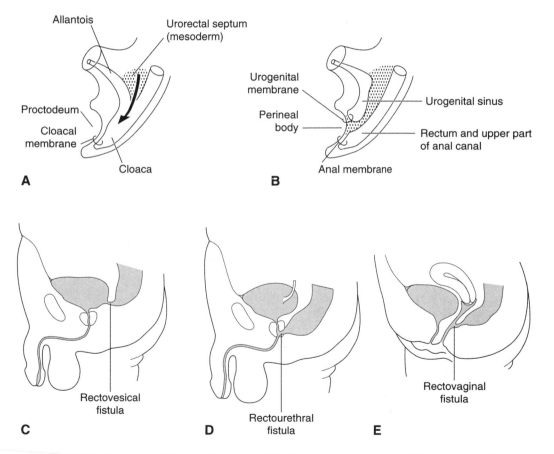

Figure 10-8. *(A)* Diagram depicting the formation of the hindgut area at week 4. *Stippled area* indicates the mesoderm making up the urorectal septum. The *bold arrow* shows the direction of growth of the urorectal septum. *(B)* At week 7. *(C, D, E)* Congenital malformations associated with the urorectal septum. *(C)* Rectovesical fistula. *(D)* Rectourethral fistula, which generally occurs in males associated with the prostatic urethra, and is sometimes called a rectoprostatic fistula. *(E)* Rectovaginal fistula. *(C-E,* Redrawn from Larsen WJ: *Human Embryology,* 2nd ed. New York, Churchill Livingstone, 1997, p. 268.)

2. The terminal end of the hindgut is an endoderm-lined pouch called the **cloaca**, which contacts the surface ectoderm of the **proctodeum** to form the **cloacal membrane**.

   a. The cloaca is partitioned by the **urorectal septum** into the **rectum and upper anal canal** and the **urogenital sinus**.

   b. The cloacal membrane is partitioned by the urorectal septum into the **anal membrane** and **urogenital membrane**. (*Note:* The urorectal septum fuses with the cloacal membrane at the future site of the gross anatomic **perineal body**.)

B. Sources

- **Simple columnar absorptive cells** lining hindgut derivatives, **goblet cells**, and **enteroendocrine cells** comprising the intestinal glands are derived from endoderm.
- Lamina propria, muscularis mucosae, submucosa, inner circular and outer longitudinal (taeniae coli) smooth muscle of the muscularis externa, and serosa are derived from visceral mesoderm.

C. Clinical considerations: Colonic aganglionosis (Hirschsprung's disease)

- results from failure of neural crest cells to form the myenteric plexus of the sigmoid colon and rectum.
- results in a loss of peristalsis in the colon segment distal to the normal innervated colon. Patients present with fecal retention and abdominal distention.
- Other congenital malformations are rare.

V. Anal Canal (Figure 10-9)

A. Development

1. The **upper anal canal** develops from the **hindgut**.

2. The **lower anal canal** develops from the **proctodeum**, which is an invagination of surface ectoderm caused by a proliferation of mesoderm surrounding the anal membrane. (*Note:* The lower anal canal is not a hindgut derivative.)

   - The dual components (hindgut and proctodeum) involved in the embryologic formation of the entire anal canal determine the gross anatomy of this area, which becomes important when considering the characteristics and metastasis of anorectal tumors.

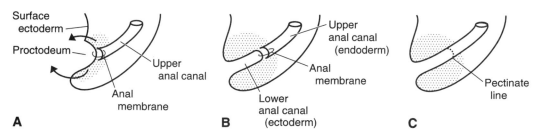

Figure 10-9. *(A, B, C)* Various stages in the formation of the anal canal. *Stippled area* indicates the mesoderm proliferations, and *curved arrows* indicate its direction of growth as it forms the lower anal canal.

3. The junction between the upper and lower anal canals is indicated by the **pectinate line**, which also marks the site of the former **anal membrane**.

B. Sources

– The **simple columnar epithelium** lining the upper anal canal is derived from endoderm, whereas the **stratified squamous epithelium** lining the lower anal canal is derived from ectoderm.

– The lamina propria, muscularis mucosae, submucosa, muscularis externa consisting of the internal and external anal sphincters, and adventitia are derived from mesoderm.

C. Clinical considerations

1. Imperforate anus

– occurs when the anal membrane fails to perforate; a layer of tissue separates the anal canal from the exterior.

2. Anal agenesis

– occurs when the anal canal ends as a blind sac **below the puborectalis muscle** due to abnormal formation of the urorectal septum.

– is usually associated with an abnormal communication between the rectum and urinary bladder (**rectovesical fistula**), rectum and urethra (**recto-urethral fistula**), or rectum and vagina (**rectovaginal fistula**).

– is associated clinically with presence of **meconium** in the urine or vagina.

3. Anorectal agenesis

– occurs when the rectum ends as a blind sac **above the puborectalis muscle** due to abnormal formation of the urorectal septum.

– is the most common type of anorectal malformation.

– is usually associated with a **rectovesical, rectourethral,** or **rectovaginal fistula**.

– is associated clinically with the presence of meconium in urine or vagina.

4. Rectal atresia

– occurs when both the rectum and anal canal are present but remain unconnected due to either abnormal recanalization or a compromised blood supply causing focal atresia.

VI. Mesenteries

– The primitive gut tube is suspended within the peritoneal cavity of the embryo by the ventral mesentery and dorsal mesentery, from which all adult mesenteries are derived (Table 10-2).

Table 10-2. Derivation of Adult Mesenteries

Embryonic Mesentery	Adult Mesentery
Ventral	Lesser omentum (hepatoduodenal and hepatogastric ligaments), falciform ligament of liver, coronary ligament of liver, triangular ligament of liver
Dorsal	Greater omentum (gastrorenal, gastrosplenic, gastrocolic, and splenorenal ligaments), mesentery of small intestine, mesoappendix, transverse mesocolon, sigmoid mesocolon

Review Test

Directions: Each of the numbered items or incomplete statements in this section is followed by answers or by completions of the statement. Select the **one** lettered answer or completion that is **best** in each case.

1. Pancreatic islets consist of alpha, beta, and delta cells, which secrete glucagon, insulin, and somatostatin, respectively. These cells are derived from

(A) mesoderm
(B) endoderm
(C) ectoderm
(D) neuroectoderm
(E) neural crest cells

2. A 2-month-old baby with severe jaundice also has dark-colored urine (deep yellow) and white clay-colored stool. Which of the following disorders might be suspected?

(A) esophageal stenosis
(B) annular pancreas
(C) hypertrophic pyloric stenosis
(D) extrahepatic biliary atresia
(E) duodenal atresia

3. A 28-day-old baby is brought to the physician because of projectile vomiting after feeding. Until this time, the baby has had no problems in feeding. On examination, a small knot is palpated at the right costal margin. Which of the following disorders might be suspected?

(A) esophageal stenosis
(B) annular pancreas
(C) hypertrophic pyloric stenosis
(D) extrahepatic biliary atresia
(E) duodenal atresia

4. Which of the following arteries supplies foregut derivatives of the digestive system?

(A) celiac trunk
(B) superior mesenteric artery
(C) inferior mesenteric artery
(D) right umbilical artery
(E) intercostal artery

5. The most common type of anorectal malformation is

(A) imperforate anus
(B) anal agenesis
(C) anorectal agenesis
(D) rectal atresia
(E) colonic aganglionosis

6. The simple columnar or cuboidal epithelium lining the extrahepatic biliary ducts is derived from

(A) mesoderm
(B) endoderm
(C) ectoderm
(D) neuroectoderm
(E) neural crest cells

7. A 4-day-old baby boy has not defecated since coming home from the hospital even though feeding has been normal without any excessive vomiting. Rectal examination reveals a normal anus, anal canal, and rectum. However, a large fecal mass is found in the colon, and a large release of flatus and feces follows the rectal examination. Which of the following conditions would be suspected?

(A) imperforate anus
(B) anal agenesis
(C) anorectal agenesis
(D) rectal atresia
(E) colonic aganglionosis

8. Which one of the following structures is derived from the midgut?

(A) appendix
(B) stomach
(C) liver
(D) pancreas
(E) sigmoid colon

9. A 3-month-old baby girl presents with a swollen umbilicus that has failed to heal normally. The umbilicus drains secretions, and there is passage of fecal material through the umbilicus at times. What is the most likely diagnosis?

(A) omphalocele
(B) gastroschisis
(C) anal agenesis
(D) ileal diverticulum
(E) intestinal stenosis

10. The midgut loop normally herniates through the primitive umbilical ring into the extraembryonic coelom during week 6 of development. Failure of the intestinal loops to return to the abdominal cavity by week 11 results in the formation of

(A) omphalocele
(B) gastroschisis
(C) anal agenesis
(D) ileal diverticulum
(E) intestinal stenosis

11. Kupffer cells present in the adult liver are derived from

(A) mesoderm
(B) endoderm
(C) ectoderm
(D) neuroectoderm
(E) neural crest cells

12. The simple columnar and stratified columnar epithelia lining the lower part of the anal canal are derived from

(A) mesoderm
(B) endoderm
(C) ectoderm
(D) neuroectoderm
(E) neural crest cells

13. A baby born to a young woman whose pregnancy was complicated by polyhydramnios was placed in the intensive care unit because of repeated vomiting containing bile. The stomach was markedly distended, and only small amounts of meconium had passed through the anus. What is the most likely diagnosis?

(A) esophageal stenosis
(B) annular pancreas
(C) hypertrophic pyloric stenosis
(D) extrahepatic biliary atresia
(E) duodenal atresia

Answers and Explanations

1–B. Pancreatic islets form as isolated clumps of cells that bud from endodermal tubules.

2–D. The baby is suffering from extrahepatic biliary atresia, which results from failure of the bile ducts to recanalize during development. This prevents bile from entering the duodenum.

3–C. The baby is suffering from hypertrophic pyloric stenosis. This occurs when the smooth muscle in the pyloric region of the stomach hypertrophies and obstructs passage of food. The hypertrophied muscle can be palpated at the right costal margin. The exact cause of this condition is not known.

4–A. The artery that supplies foregut derivatives of the digestive system is the celiac trunk. The celiac trunk consists of the left gastric artery, splenic artery, and common hepatic artery. The superior mesenteric artery supplies the midgut, and the inferior mesenteric artery supplies the hindgut.

5–C. The most common type of malformation involving the anal canal and rectum is anorectal agenesis, in which the rectum ends as a blind sac above the puborectalis muscle. The anal canal may form normally but does not connect with the rectum. This malformation is accompanied by various fistulas.

6–B. The epithelium lining the extrahepatic biliary ducts is derived from endoderm. The intrahepatic biliary ducts are also derived from endoderm.

7–E. This baby boy suffers from colonic aganglionosis, or Hirschsprung's disease, which results in the retention of fecal material, causing the normal colon to enlarge. The retention of fecal material results from a lack of peristalsis in the narrow segment of colon distal to the enlarged colon. A biopsy of the narrow segment of colon would reveal the absence of parasympathetic ganglion cells in the myenteric plexus caused by failure of neural crest migration.

8–A. The appendix is derived from the midgut. The midgut normally undergoes a 270° counterclockwise rotation during development; malrotation of the midgut may result in the appendix lying in the upper part of the abdominal cavity, which may affect a diagnosis of appendicitis.

9–D. This baby girl has an ileal diverticulum (Meckel's diverticulum), which occurs when a remnant of the vitelline duct persists. In this case, a fistula is present whereby contents of the ileum can be discharged onto the surface of the skin.

10–A. An omphalocele results when intestinal loops fail to return to the abdominal cavity. Instead, the intestinal loops remain in the umbilical cord covered by amnion.

11–A. Kupffer cells are actually macrophages and are derived from mesoderm. Hepatocytes and the epithelial lining of the intrahepatic biliary tree are derived from endoderm.

12–C. The anal canal is formed from two components, the hindgut and proctodeum. The epithelium lining the lower anal canal is derived from ectoderm lining the proctodeum.

13–E. This baby is suffering from duodenal atresia at a level distal to the opening of the common bile duct. This causes a reflux of bile and its presence in the vomitus. The pregnancy was complicated by polyhydramnios because the duodenal atresia prevented passage of amniotic fluid into the intestines for absorption.

11

Respiratory System

I. Upper Respiratory System

– consists of the **nose, nasopharynx,** and **oropharynx.**

– is discussed in Chapter 12.

II. Lower Respiratory System (Figure 11-1)

– consists of the **larynx, trachea, bronchi,** and **lungs.**

A. Early development

– The first sign of development is the formation of the **laryngotracheal diverticulum** in the ventral wall of the primitive foregut during week 4.

– The distal end of the laryngotracheal diverticulum enlarges to form the **lung bud.**

– The laryngotracheal diverticulum initially is in open communication with the foregut, but eventually they become separated by folds of mesoderm, the **tracheoesophageal folds.**

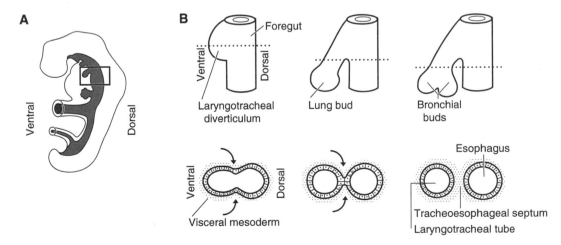

Figure 11-1. Early development of respiratory system. *(A)* Lateral view of an embryo at day 25, showing the entire primitive gut tube. The area in the rectangle indicates the portion of foregut involved in respiratory development. This area is enlarged in *B.* *(B)* Relationship of the laryngotracheal diverticulum and foregut. Curved arrows indicate the movement of the tracheoesophageal folds as the tracheoesophageal septum forms between the future trachea and esophagus.

139

– When the tracheoesophageal folds fuse in the midline to form the **tracheoesophageal septum**, the primitive foregut is divided into the **laryngotracheal tube** ventrally and **esophagus** dorsally.

B. Development of the larynx

– The opening of the laryngotracheal diverticulum into the primitive foregut becomes the **laryngeal orifice**.
– Laryngeal **epithelium** and **glands** are derived from **endoderm**.
– **Laryngeal muscles** are derived from **somitomeric mesoderm of pharyngeal arches 4 and 6** and therefore are innervated by the **superior laryngeal nerve** and **recurrent laryngeal nerve,** which are branches of CN X.
– **Laryngeal connective tissue** and **cartilages** (thyroid, cricoid, arytenoid, corniculate, and cuneiform) are derived from **mesoderm** of pharyngeal arches 4 and 6.

C. Development of the trachea

1. Sources

– **Tracheal epithelium** and **glands** are derived from **endoderm**.
– **Tracheal smooth muscle, connective tissue,** and **C-shaped cartilage rings** are derived from **mesoderm**.

2. Clinical considerations

a. Tracheoesophageal fistula (Figure 11-2)

– is an abnormal communication (**fistula**) between the trachea and esophagus.
– is generally associated with **esophageal atresia** and **polyhydramnios**.
– results from improper division of foregut by the tracheoesophageal septum.
– Five anatomic types have been described; the most common (85%–90% of all cases) is **esophageal atresia with a fistula between distal end of esophagus and trachea**.

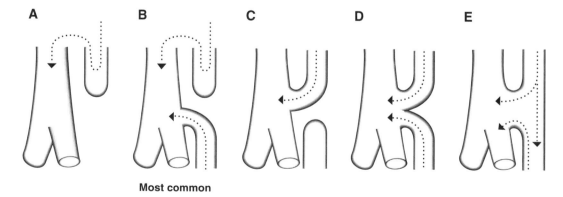

Most common

Figure 11-2. Five different anatomic types of esophagus and trachea malformation. *(A)* Esophageal atresia only. *(B)* Esophageal atresia with a tracheoesophageal fistula at distal end; most common type, occurring in 85%–90% of cases. *(C)* Esophageal atresia with a tracheoesophageal fistula at proximal end. *(D)* Esophageal atresia with a tracheoesophageal fistula at proximal and distal end. *(E)* Tracheoesophageal fistula only. Dotted lines and arrows indicate possible directions of flow of contents.

- Clinical features include **excessive accumulation of saliva or mucus** in the nose and mouth; episodes of **gagging and cyanosis** after swallowing milk; **abdominal distention after crying**; and **reflux of gastric contents into lungs, causing pneumonitis**.
- Diagnostic features include **inability to pass a catheter** into the stomach and x-rays demonstrating **air in the infant's stomach**.

b. Tracheal stenosis and atresia

- are rare malformations in which narrowing (stenosis) or closure (atresia) of the tracheal lumen is observed.
- are usually associated with a tracheoesophageal fistula.

c. Tracheal diverticulum

- is a rare malformation in which a blind bronchus-like projection occurs off the trachea.

D. Development of the bronchi

1. Stages of development (Figure 11-3)

- The lung bud divides into two **bronchial buds**.
- In week 5 of development, bronchial buds enlarge to form **primary bronchi**; the right primary bronchus is larger and more vertical than the left primary bronchus; this relationship persists throughout adult life and accounts for the greater likelihood of foreign bodies lodging on the right side than on the left.
- Primary bronchi further subdivide into **secondary bronchi** (three on the right side and two on the left, corresponding to the lobes of the lung).
- Secondary bronchi further subdivide into **tertiary, or segmental, bronchi** (10 on the right side and 8–9 on the left). These are the primordia of the **bronchopulmonary segments**.
- As the bronchi develop, they expand laterally and caudally into a space known as the **primitive pleural cavity**; visceral mesoderm covering the outside of the bronchi develops into **visceral pleura**, and **somatic**

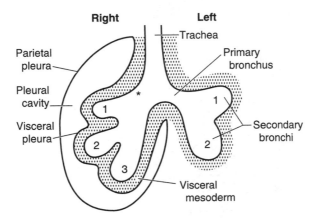

Figure 11-3. Later development of respiratory system. The right primary bronchus is larger and more vertical than the left (see *asterisk* [*]). The relationship of the lung and pleural cavity can best be appreciated by visualizing the pleura and pleural cavity as a balloon. The wall of the balloon in apposition to the lung is visceral pleura and that lining the body wall is parietal pleura. As the prolific growth of the lung continues, the balloon is squeezed to its adult slit-like form, with visceral pleura almost in contact with parietal pleura.

mesoderm covering the inside of the body wall develops into **parietal pleura**.

2. Sources

- **Bronchial epithelium and glands** are derived from **endoderm**.
- **Bronchial smooth muscle, connective tissue**, and **cartilage** are derived from **visceral mesoderm**.

3. Clinical considerations

a. Bronchopulmonary segment

- is a segment of lung tissue supplied by a tertiary (segmental) bronchus.
- Surgeons can resect diseased lung tissue along bronchopulmonary segments rather than removing the entire lobe.

b. Congenital neonatal emphysema

- is an overdistention with air of one or more lobes of the lung.
- is caused by collapsed bronchi due to failure of bronchial cartilage development.
- Air can be inspired through collapsed bronchi but cannot be expired.

c. Congenital bronchial cysts (bronchiectasis)

- are caused by dilation of bronchi.
- Cysts may be solitary or multiple, filled with air or fluid.
- Multiple cysts demonstrate a honeycomb appearance on x-rays.

E. Development of the lungs

1. Periods of development (Figure 11-4)

- Time periods overlap because the lung matures in a **proximal–distal direction**, beginning with the largest bronchi and proceeding outward.
- As a result, lung development is **heterogeneous**; proximal pulmonary tissue will be in a more advanced period of development than distal pulmonary tissue.

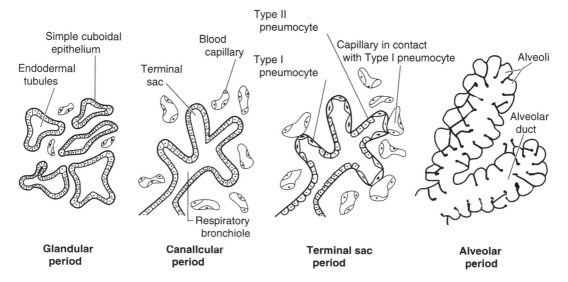

Figure 11-4. Four time periods of lung development as described histologically.

a. Glandular period (weeks 5–17)

- Developing lung resembles branching of a compound exocrine gland into a bush-like array of endodermal tubules, which comprise the air-conducting system.
- Histologic structures involved in gas exchange are not yet formed, and respiration is not possible.
- Premature fetuses born during this period cannot survive.

b. Canalicular period (weeks 13–25)

- **Respiratory bronchioles** and **terminal sacs** (primitive alveoli) develop.
- Vascularization increases due to capillaries forming in visceral mesoderm surrounding the respiratory bronchioles and terminal sacs.
- **Premature fetuses born at less than 20 weeks' gestation rarely survive.**

c. Terminal sac period (week 24–birth)

- The number of terminal sacs and vascularization increases greatly.
- Differentiation of **Type I pneumocytes** (thin, flat cells that make up part of the blood–air barrier) and **Type II pneumocytes** (which produce **surfactant**) begins.
- Capillaries make contact with Type I pneumocytes, which permits respiration.
- **Premature fetuses born between week 25 and week 28 can survive with intensive care; this is the earliest period at which fetuses can survive.**
- Adequate vascularization and surfactant levels are the most important factors for the survival of premature infants.

d. Alveolar period (week 29–age 8 years)

- Lung development continues after birth until about **age 8 years**.
- By age 8, the adult complement of 300 million alveoli is reached.
- Increase in size of lung after birth is caused by the increased number of respiratory bronchioles and terminal sacs.
- Terminal sacs develop into mature alveolar ducts and alveoli.
- Histologically a mature **blood–air barrier** derived from **visceral mesoderm and endoderm** is established.
- On chest x-rays, lungs of a newborn infant are **denser** than an adult lung because of the fewer number of mature alveoli.

2. Clinical considerations

a. Aeration at birth

- is the replacement of fluid with air in the newborn's lungs.
- At birth, lungs are half-filled with fluid derived from the lungs (main source), amniotic cavity, and tracheal glands.
- Fluid is eliminated at birth through nose and mouth during delivery, and through resorption by pulmonary capillaries and lymphatics.
- Lungs of a stillborn baby will sink when placed in water because they contain fluid rather than air.

b. Respiratory distress syndrome (RDS)

- is caused by a deficiency or absence of **surfactant**, a surface-active detergent composed of **phosphatidylcholine (mainly dipalmitoyl lecithin) and proteins**, which coats the inside of alveoli and maintains alveolar patency.
- **Thyroxine** and **cortisol** increase production of surfactant.
- Prolonged intrauterine asphyxia decreases production of surfactant by permanently damaging Type II pneumocytes.
- is common in **premature infants** and **infants of diabetic mothers**.
- accounts for 50%–70% of deaths in premature infants.
- not only threatens the infant with immediate asphyxiation, but also can bring about **hyaline membrane disease**, repeated gasping inhalations can damage the alveolar lining and cause hyaline membrane disease.
- Hyaline membrane disease is characterized histologically by collapsed alveoli (atelectasis) containing an eosinophilic fluid that resembles a hyaline or glassy membrane.

c. Pulmonary agenesis

- is complete absence of lungs, bronchi, and vasculature.
- is a rare condition caused by failure of bronchial buds to develop.
- Unilateral pulmonary agenesis is compatible with life.

d. Pulmonary hypoplasia

- is a poorly developed bronchial tree with abnormal histology.
- can be found in association with **congenital diaphragmatic hernia**; herniation of abdominal contents into the thorax compresses the developing lung.
- can be found in association with **bilateral renal agenesis**, which causes an insufficient amount of amniotic fluid (**oligohydramnios**) to be produced, which in turn increases pressure on the fetal thorax.
- may be partial (involving a small segment of lung) or total (entire lung).

Review Test

Directions: Each of the numbered items or incomplete statements in this section is followed by answers or by completions of the statement. Select the **one** lettered answer or completion that is **best** in each case.

1. All of the following findings would indicate a diagnosis of tracheoesophageal fistula with esophageal atresia EXCEPT

(A) excessive saliva and mucus
(B) abdominal distention after crying
(C) regurgitation after feeding
(D) oligohydramnios during pregnancy
(E) reflux of gastric contents into lungs

2. Within hours after birth, a baby, whose mother is diabetic, had a rising respiratory rate and labored breathing. The baby became cyanotic and died. Postmortem histologic examination revealed collapsed alveoli lined with eosinophilic material. What is the diagnosis?

(A) congenital emphysema
(B) respiratory distress syndrome
(C) cystic fibrosis
(D) tracheoesophageal fistula
(E) pulmonary carcinoma

3. The trachea is lined with pseudostratified ciliated columnar epithelium with goblet cells. This epithelium is derived from

(A) neuroectoderm
(B) endoderm
(C) ectoderm
(D) visceral mesoderm
(E) mesoderm of fourth and sixth pharyngeal arches

4. Smooth muscle, connective tissue, and cartilage of primary bronchi are derived from which of the following sources?

(A) neuroectoderm
(B) endoderm
(C) ectoderm
(D) visceral mesoderm
(E) mesoderm of pharyngeal arches 4 and 6

5. Components of the blood–air barrier in the lung are derived from which of the following sources?

(A) ectoderm only
(B) visceral mesoderm only
(C) visceral mesoderm and ectoderm
(D) endoderm and ectoderm
(E) visceral mesoderm and endoderm

6. The laryngotracheal tube initially is in open communication with the primitive foregut. Which of the following embryonic structures is responsible for separating these two structures?

(A) laryngotracheal groove
(B) posterior esophageal folds
(C) laryngotracheal diverticulum
(D) tracheoesophageal septum
(E) bronchopulmonary segment

7. Collapsed bronchi caused by failure of bronchial cartilage development is indicative of which one of the following congenital malformations?

(A) congenital bronchial cysts
(B) congenital neonatal emphysema
(C) tracheoesophageal fistula
(D) hyaline membrane disease
(E) pulmonary hypoplasia

8. Pulmonary hypoplasia is commonly associated with which condition?

(A) hyaline membrane disease
(B) diaphragmatic hernia
(C) tracheoesophageal fistula
(D) congenital bronchial cysts
(E) congenital neonatal emphysema

9. Development of which of the following is the first sign of respiratory system development?

(A) tracheoesophageal septum
(B) hypobranchial eminence
(C) primitive foregut
(D) tracheoesophageal fistula
(E) laryngotracheal diverticulum

Directions: Each group of items in this section consists of lettered options followed by a set of numbered items. For each item, select the **one** lettered option that is most closely associated with it. Each lettered option may be selected once, more than once, or not at all.

Questions 10–16

Match each statement concerning lung development with the appropriate time period.

(A) Week 4 of gestation
(B) Weeks 5–17 of gestation
(C) Weeks 13–25 of gestation
(D) Week 24 of gestation to birth
(E) Weeks 25–28 of gestation
(F) Age 8 years

10. Earliest period at which premature fetuses typically survive

11. Canalicular period

12. Development of respiratory system begins

13. Development of respiratory system ends

14. Glandular period

15. Differentiation of Type I and Type II pneumocytes begins

16. Majority of mature alveoli are formed

Answers and Explanations

1–D. Oligohydramnios is a low volume of amniotic fluid (400 ml in third trimester). Polyhydramnios is an excessive volume of amniotic fluid and occurs when the fetus cannot swallow the usual amount of amniotic fluid, as in esophageal atresia.

2–B. Respiratory distress syndrome is common in premature infants and infants of diabetic mothers. It is caused by a deficiency or absence of surfactant. Collapsed alveoli and eosinophilic material consisting of fibrin (hyaline membrane) can be observed histologically, indicating associated hyaline membrane disease.

3–B. The epithelial lining of the entire respiratory system (from tracheal epithelium to Type I pneumocytes lining alveoli) is derived from endoderm.

4–D. The epithelium of primary bronchi is derived from endoderm; the other components are derived from visceral mesoderm.

5–E. The blood–air barrier comprises the structures through which gaseous exchange occurs between air in alveoli and blood in pulmonary capillaries. The attenuated pulmonary epithelium (Type I pneumocytes) is derived from endoderm. The simple, squamous epithelium (endothelium) lining pulmonary capillaries is derived from visceral mesoderm.

6–D. When the tracheoesophageal folds fuse in the midline, they form the tracheoesophageal septum. This septum is responsible for separating the adult trachea ventrally from the esophagus dorsally.

7–B. Congenital neonatal emphysema is a malformation involving the bronchi. One or more lobes of the lungs are overdistended with air because air can be inspired through collapsed bronchi, but cannot be expired.

8–B. During normal development, a space is provided for the prolific growth of the bronchial buds in a lateral and caudal direction. This space, which is part of the intraembryonic coelom, is called the primitive pleural cavity. If this space is reduced by herniation of abdominal viscera, lung development will be severely compromised.

9–E. Development of the respiratory system begins in week 4; the first sign of development is formation of the laryngotracheal diverticulum in the ventral wall of the primitive foregut.

10–E. The earliest age at which premature fetuses typically survive is between weeks 25 and 28 of gestation (weighing about 1000 g). These weeks fall within the terminal sac period (week 24–birth), when adequate vascularization and surfactant levels are in the process of being reached. If a baby is born prematurely, the state of lung development is usually the prime factor in determining whether the child will live or die.

11–C. The canalicular period is between weeks 13 and 25 of gestation. During this time, respiratory bronchioles and terminal sacs develop, but premature fetuses born during this period usually die.

12–A. The embryonic period is between weeks 3 and 8 of development. During this time, formation of all basic organ systems, including the respiratory system, begins. The laryngotracheal diverticulum (first sign of lung development) can be observed in the ventral wall of the primitive foregut at week 4.

13–F. Lung development continues after birth until age 8 years. During these 8 years, the increase in lung size is due to an increased number of respiratory bronchioles and terminal sacs.

14–B. The glandular period is between weeks 5 and 17 of gestation. During this time, respiration is not possible and premature fetuses cannot survive.

15–D. Type I pneumocytes (components of the blood–air barrier) and Type II pneumocytes (which produce surfactant) begin to differentiate during the terminal sac period.

16–F. Lung development continues after birth until age 8 years. At birth, only about 12%–16% of the adult number of mature alveoli are present. The adult complement of 300 million alveoli is reached by age 8.

12

Head and Neck

I. Pharyngeal Apparatus (Figure 12-1)

- contributes greatly to the formation of the head and neck.
- consists of **pharyngeal arches, pharyngeal pouches, pharyngeal grooves,** and **pharyngeal membranes**.
- is first observed in week 4 of development and gives the embryo its distinctive appearance.

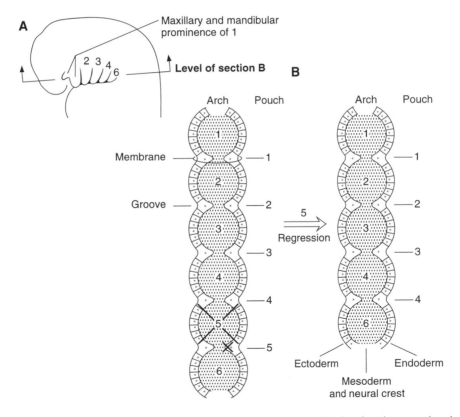

Figure 12-1. *(A)* Lateral view of an embryo in week 4 of development, showing the pharyngeal arches. Note that pharyngeal arch 1 consists of a maxillary prominence and a mandibular prominence, which can cause some confusion in numbering of the arches. *(B)* A schematic diagram indicating a convenient way to understand the numbering of the arches and pouches. The *X*'s indicate regression of pharyngeal arch and pouch 5.

– There are five pharyngeal arches (1, 2, 3, 4, and 6) and four pharyngeal pouches (1, 2, 3, and 4), four pharyngeal grooves (1, 2, 3, and 4), and four pharyngeal membranes (1, 2, 3, and 4).

– Pharyngeal arch 5 and pharyngeal pouch 5 completely regress in the human. Aortic arch 5 also completely regresses (see Chapter 5).

A. Pharyngeal arches

1. Makeup of the pharyngeal arches

– Arches consist of **somitomeric mesoderm** (from somitomeres 1–7; see Chapter 4) and **neural crest cells**.

– Each pharyngeal arch has a **cranial nerve** associated with it.

a. Somitomeric mesoderm differentiates into an **artery** (aortic arches 1–6) and **muscle tissue**.

b. Neural crest differentiates into **skeletal components** and **connective tissue**. Neural crest cells can differentiate into nonneural components.

2. Fate of the pharyngeal arches (Table 12-1)

Table 12-1. Adult Derivatives of the Pharyngeal Arches

Arch*	Nerve	Adult Derivatives	
		Mesoderm	**Neural Crest Cells**
1	CN V	Muscles of mastication, mylohyoid muscle, tensor veli palatini muscle, tensor tympani muscle, anterior belly of the digastric muscle	Maxilla, zygomatic bone, squamous temporal bone, palatine bone, vomer, mandible, incus, malleus, sphenomandibular ligament
2	CN VII	Muscles of facial expression, posterior belly of the digastric muscle, stylohyoid muscle, stapedius muscle	Lesser horn and upper body of hyoid bone, stapes, styloid process, stylohyoid ligament
3	CN IX	Stylopharyngeus muscle	Greater horn and lower body of hyoid bone
4	CN X (superior laryngeal branch)	Muscles of the soft palate (except tensor veli palatini), muscles of the pharynx (except stylopharyngeus), cricothyroid muscle, cricopharyngeus muscle, laryngeal cartilages	...
6	CN X (recurrent laryngeal branch)	Intrinsic muscles of the larynx (except cricothyroid), upper muscles of esophagus, laryngeal cartilages	...

* The arteries associated with the arches (aortic arches) have been discussed in Chapter 5.
Reprinted from Dudek RW: *High-Yield Embryology*. Baltimore, Williams & Wilkins, 1996, p. 30.

B. **Pharyngeal pouches** (Figure 12-2)

1. Makeup of the pharyngeal pouches: They are diverticula (pouches) of the endodermal lining of the **foregut**.

2. Fate of the pharyngeal pouches (Table 12-2)

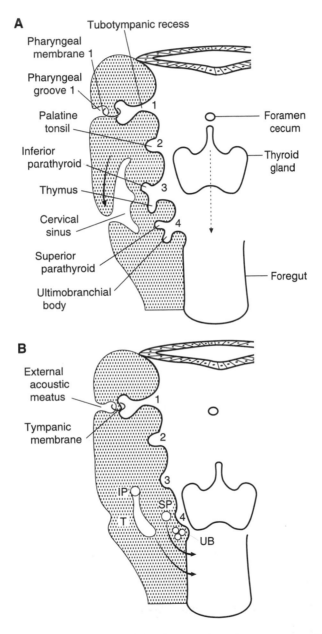

Figure 12-2. Schematic diagrams of the fate of the pharyngeal pouches, grooves, and membranes. *(A) Solid arrow* indicates the downward growth of pharyngeal arch 2, thereby forming a smooth contour at the neck region. *Dotted arrow* indicates downward migration of the thyroid gland. *(B) Curved arrows* indicate direction of migration of the inferior parathyroid (IP), thymus (T), superior parathyroid (SP), and ultimobranchial bodies (UB). Note that the parathyroid tissue derived from pharyngeal pouch 3 is carried farther caudally by the descent of the thymus than parathyroid tissue from pharyngeal pouch 4.

Table 12-2. Adult Derivatives of the Pharyngeal Pouches

Pouch	Adult Derivatives
1	Epithelial lining of auditory tube and middle ear cavity
2	Epithelial lining of palatine tonsil crypts
3	Inferior parathyroid gland, thymus
4	Superior parathyroid gland, ultimobranchial body*

* Neural crest cells migrate into the ultimobranchial body to form the C-cells (calcitonin secreting cells) of the thyroid.
Reprinted from Dudek RW: *High-Yield Embryology.* Baltimore, Williams & Wilkins, 1996, p. 30.

C. Pharyngeal grooves

1. Makeup of the pharyngeal grooves: They are the invaginations of ectoderm between each pharyngeal arch.

2. Fate of the pharyngeal grooves

   a. Pharyngeal groove 1 gives rise to the **external acoustic meatus**.

   b. The other grooves are obliterated as pharyngeal arch 2 overgrows pharyngeal arches 3 and 4.

D. Pharyngeal membranes

1. Makeup of the pharyngeal membranes: They are structures consisting of ectoderm, intervening mesoderm and neural crest, and endoderm between each pharyngeal arch.

2. Fate of the pharyngeal membranes

   a. Pharyngeal membrane 1 gives rise to the **tympanic membrane** of the ear.

   b. The other membranes form no definitive adult structure.

II. Development of the Thyroid Gland

– In the midline of the floor of the pharynx, the endodermal lining of the foregut forms the **thyroid diverticulum**.

– The thyroid diverticulum migrates caudally, passing ventral to the hyoid bone and laryngeal cartilages.

– During this migration, the thyroid remains connected to the tongue by the **thyroglossal duct**, which later is obliterated.

– The site of the thyroglossal duct is indicated in the adult by the **foramen cecum**.

– **Follicular cells** of the thyroid are derived from endoderm.

III. Development of the Tongue (Figure 12-3)

A. Oral part (anterior two-thirds) of the tongue

1. **Formation**

   – Three mesodermal swellings, the **median tongue bud** and two **distal tongue buds**, develop in the floor of the pharynx at pharyngeal arch 1.

   – The distal tongue buds overgrow the median tongue bud and fuse in the midline, forming the **median sulcus**.

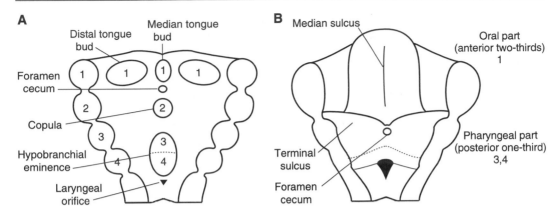

Figure 12-3. Diagram showing the development of the tongue. *(A)* At week 5. *(B)* In the newborn.

- is characterized by **filiform papillae** (no taste buds), **fungiform papillae** (taste buds present), and **circumvallate papillae** (taste buds present).

2. **Innervation**
   - General sensation from the mucosa is carried by the **lingual branch of the trigeminal nerve** (CN V).
   - Taste sensation from the mucosa is carried by the **chorda tympani branch of the facial nerve** (CN VII).

B. **Pharyngeal part (posterior one-third) of the tongue**

1. **Formation**
   - Two mesodermal swellings, the **copula** and **hypobranchial eminence**, develop in the floor of the pharynx at pharyngeal arches 2, 3, and 4.
   - The hypobranchial eminence overgrows the copula, thereby eliminating any contribution of pharyngeal arch 2 in the formation of the definitive adult tongue.
   - The line of fusion between the oral and pharyngeal parts of the tongue is indicated by the **terminal sulcus**.
   - is characterized by the lingual tonsil, which, along with the palatine tonsil and pharyngeal tonsil (adenoids), forms **Waldeyer's ring**, which protects the oral port of entry.

2. **Innervation**
   - General sensation from the mucosa is carried primarily by the **glossopharyngeal nerve** (CN IX).
   - Taste sensation from the mucosa is carried predominantly by the **glossopharyngeal nerve** (CN IX).

C. **Muscles of the tongue**
   - The intrinsic muscles and extrinsic muscles (styloglossus, hyoglossus, and genioglossus) are derived from myoblasts that migrate into the tongue region from **occipital somites**.

– Motor innervation is supplied by the **hypoglossal nerve** (CN XII), except for **palatoglossus muscle**, which is innervated by CN X.

IV. Development of the Mouth

– The mouth is formed from a surface depression called the **stomodeum**, which is lined by ectoderm, and the **cephalic end of the foregut**, which is lined by endoderm.
– The stomodeum and foregut meet at the **oropharyngeal membrane**.
– The epithelium of the **oral part of the tongue, hard palate, sides of the mouth, lips, parotid gland and ducts, Rathke's pouch,** and **enamel of the teeth** are derived from ectoderm.
– The epithelium of the **pharyngeal part of the tongue, floor of the mouth, palatoglossal fold, palatopharyngeal fold, soft palate, sublingual gland and ducts,** and **submandibular gland and ducts** are derived from endoderm.

V. Development of the Face (Figure 12-4)

– The face is formed by three swellings, the **frontonasal prominence, maxillary prominence** (pharyngeal arch 1), and **mandibular prominence** (pharyngeal arch 1).
– Bilateral ectodermal thickenings called **nasal placodes** develop on the ventrolateral aspects of the frontonasal prominence.
– The nasal placodes invaginate into the underlying mesoderm to form the **nasal pits,** thereby producing a ridge of tissue that forms the **medial and lateral nasal prominences**.

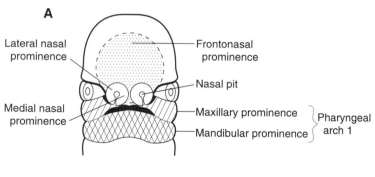

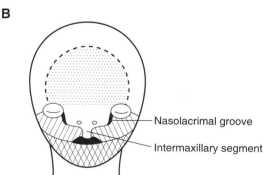

Figure 12-4. Diagram showing the development of the face. Note that pharyngeal arch 1 plays a major role. *(A)* At week 6. *(B)* At week 10.

– A deep groove—the **nasolacrimal groove**—forms between the maxillary prominence and the lateral nasal prominence and eventually forms the **nasolacrimal duct** and **lacrimal sac**.

VI. Development of the Nasal Cavities

A. The nasal placodes deepen considerably to form the nasal pits and finally the **nasal sacs**.

B. The nasal sacs remain separated from the oral cavity by the **oronasal membrane**, but it soon ruptures; the nasal cavities and oral cavity are then continuous via the **primitive choanae**.

C. Swellings in the lateral wall of each nasal cavity form the **superior, middle, and inferior conchae**.

D. In the roof of each nasal cavity, the ectoderm of the nasal placode forms a thickened patch, the **olfactory epithelium**.

    1. Olfactory epithelium contains **sustentacular cells, basal cells,** and **ciliated cells**.

    2. These ciliated cells are bipolar neurons that give rise to the **olfactory nerve** (CN I), have a life span of 1–2 months, and are continuously regenerated.

VII. Development of the Palate (Figures 12-5 and 12-6)

A. Intermaxillary segment

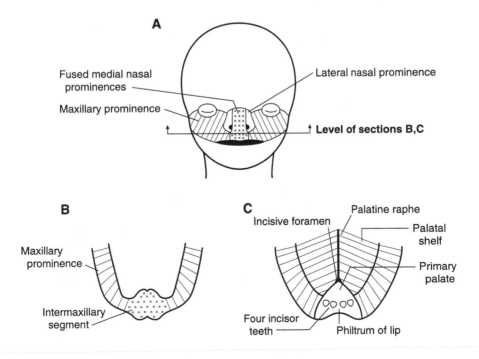

Figure 12-5. Diagram demonstrating the formation of the intermaxillary segment (*tiny X's*). (*A*) Frontal view. (*B* and *C*) Horizontal sections as indicated.

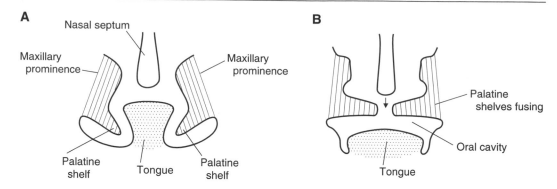

Figure 12-6. Diagram demonstrating the formation of the secondary palate. *(A)* At week 6. *(B)* At week 8.

- forms when the medial growth of the maxillary prominences causes the two medial nasal prominences to fuse together at the midline.
- consists of the **philtrum of the lip, four incisor teeth,** and the **primary palate**.

  B. **Secondary palate** (see Figures 12-5 and 12-6)

- forms from outgrowths of the maxillary prominences called the **palatine shelves**.
- Initially the palatine shelves project downward on either side of the tongue but later attain a horizontal position and fuse along the **palatine raphe** to form the **secondary palate**.
- The primary and secondary palate fuse at the **incisive foramen** to form the **definitive palate**.
- Bone develops in both the primary palate and anterior part of the secondary palate.
- Bone does not develop in the posterior part of the secondary palate, which eventually forms the **soft palate** and **uvula**.
- The **nasal septum** develops from the medial nasal prominences and fuses with the definitive palate.

VIII. Clinical Considerations

A. Pharyngeal fistula

- occurs when **pharyngeal pouch 2** and **pharyngeal groove 2 persist**, thereby forming a patent opening from the internal tonsillar area to the external neck.
- is generally found along the **anterior border of the sternocleidomastoid muscle**.

B. Pharyngeal cyst

- occurs when parts of the **pharyngeal grooves** that are normally obliterated persist, thereby forming a cyst.
- is generally found near the **angle of the mandible**.

C. First arch syndrome

– results from abnormal development of pharyngeal arch 1 and produces various facial anomalies.
– is caused by a lack of migration of **neural crest cells** into pharyngeal arch 1.
– Two well-described first arch syndromes are **Treacher Collins syndrome** and **Pierre Robin syndrome**.

D. DiGeorge syndrome

– occurs when **pharyngeal pouches 3 and 4** fail to differentiate into the thymus and parathyroid glands.
– is usually accompanied by **facial anomalies** resembling first arch syndrome and **cardiovascular anomalies** due to abnormal neural crest cell migration during formation of the aorticopulmonary septum.

E. Ectopic thymus, parathyroid, or thyroid tissue

– results from the abnormal migration of these glands from their embryonic position to their definitive adult location.
– Glandular tissue may be found anywhere along the migratory path.

F. Thyroglossal duct cyst

– occurs when parts of the thyroglossal duct persist and thereby form a cyst.
– is most commonly located in the midline near the hyoid bone, but may also be located at the base of the tongue; is then called a **lingual cyst**.

G. Ankyloglossia (tongue-tie)

– occurs when the frenulum of the tongue extends to the tip of the tongue, thereby preventing protrusion.

H. Cleft palate

– has multifactorial causes.
– is classified as anterior or posterior. (*Note:* The anatomic landmark that separates anterior from posterior cleft palate defects is the incisive foramen.)

1. Anterior cleft palate

– occurs when the palatine shelves fail to fuse with the primary palate.

2. Posterior cleft palate

– occurs when the palatine shelves fail to fuse with each other and with the nasal septum.

3. Anteroposterior cleft palate

– occurs when there is a combination of both defects.

I. Cleft lip

– has multifactorial causes. (*Note:* Cleft lip and cleft palate are distinct malformations based on their embryologic formation, even though they often occur together.)
– may occur unilaterally or bilaterally. **Unilateral cleft lip** is the most common congenital malformation of the head and neck.

– results from the following:

1. The maxillary prominence fails to fuse with the medial nasal prominence.

2. The underlying somitomeric mesoderm and neural crest fail to expand, resulting in a **persistent labial groove**.

Review Test

Directions: Each of the numbered items or incomplete statements in this section is followed by answers or by completions of the statement. Select the **one** lettered answer or completion that is **best** in each case.

1. The most common site of a thyroglossal cyst is

(A) dorsal aspect of neck
(B) anterior border of sternocleidomastoid muscle
(C) superior mediastinum
(D) midline close to the hyoid bone
(E) base of the tongue

2. Taste sensation from the oral part (anterior two-thirds) of the tongue is predominantly carried by

(A) trigeminal nerve (CN V)
(B) chorda tympani branch of the facial nerve (CN VII)
(C) glossopharyngeal nerve (CN IX)
(D) superior laryngeal branch of the vagus nerve (CN X)
(E) recurrent laryngeal branch of the vagus nerve (CN X)

3. The intermaxillary segment forms via the fusion of the

(A) maxillary prominences
(B) mandibular prominences
(C) palatine shelves
(D) lateral nasal prominences
(E) medial nasal prominences

4. The most common site of a pharyngeal fistula is the

(A) dorsal aspect of neck
(B) anterior border of sternocleidomastoid muscle
(C) superior mediastinum
(D) midline close to the hyoid bone
(E) base of the tongue

5. What is the most common congenital malformation of the head and neck region?

(A) anterior cleft palate
(B) posterior cleft palate
(C) thyroglossal duct cyst
(D) unilateral cleft lip
(E) ankyloglossia

6. Which pharyngeal arch is associated with Treacher Collins syndrome?

(A) pharyngeal arch 1
(B) pharyngeal arch 2
(C) pharyngeal arch 3
(D) pharyngeal arch 4
(E) pharyngeal arch 6

7. During surgery for the removal of a thyroid tumor, a number of small masses of glandular tissue are noted just lateral to the thyroid gland. Metastasis from the thyroid tumor is suspected, but histologic analysis of a biopsy reveals parathyroid tissue and remnants of thymus. How can this finding be explained?

(A) tumor tissue has differentiated into normal tissue
(B) a parathyroid gland tumor is also present
(C) ectopic glandular tissue is commonly found in this region
(D) patient has DiGeorge syndrome
(E) the glandular tissue is a result of a thyroglossal duct cyst

Directions: Each group of items in this section consists of lettered options followed by a set of numbered items. For each item, select the **one** lettered option that is most closely associated with it. Each lettered option may be selected once, more than once, or not at all.

Questions 8–19

For each of the following structures, select the most appropriate pharyngeal arch or pharyngeal pouch.

(A) Pharyngeal arch 1
(B) Pharyngeal arch 2
(C) Pharyngeal arch 3
(D) Pharyngeal arch 4
(E) Pharyngeal arch 6
(F) Pharyngeal pouch 1
(G) Pharyngeal pouch 2
(H) Pharyngeal pouch 3
(I) Pharyngeal pouch 4

8. Inferior parathyroid gland

9. Muscles of facial expression

10. Ultimobranchial body

11. Middle ear cavity

12. Glossopharyngeal nerve (CN IX)

13. Muscles of mastication

14. Maxilla

15. Thymus

16. Palatine tonsil

17. Facial nerve (CN VII)

18. Constrictor muscles of the pharynx

19. Intrinsic muscles of the larynx

Answers and Explanations

1–D. The thyroid gland forms from a diverticulum in the midline of the floor of the pharynx. The thyroid migrates caudally and passes ventral to the hyoid bone. During this migration, the thyroid remains connected to the tongue by the thyroglossal duct. If a part of the thyroglossal duct persists, a cyst will develop, usually near the hyoid bone.

2–B. Taste sensation from the mucosa for the oral part of the tongue is carried by the chorda tympani branch of the facial nerve (CN VII). This part of the tongue forms from pharyngeal arch 1, so the trigeminal nerve (CN V) will carry sensory innervation from the mucosa.

3–E. The intermaxillary segment, which plays a critical role in the formation of the definitive adult palate, forms when the two medial nasal prominences fuse in the midline.

4–B. A pharyngeal fistula forms when pharyngeal pouch 2 and pharyngeal groove 2 persist. Therefore, these fistulas are found on the lateral aspect of the neck, usually along the anterior border of the sternocleidomastoid muscle.

5–D. Unilateral cleft lip is the most common congenital malformation of the head and neck. Cleft lip occurs when the maxillary prominences fail to fuse with the medial nasal prominences and when the underlying somitomeric mesoderm and neural crest fail to proliferate, resulting in a persistent labial groove. Cleft lip occurs in 1 out of 900 births and may be unilateral or bilateral.

6–A. First arch syndrome results from abnormal development of pharyngeal arch 1 due to a lack of migration of neural crest cells. Treacher Collins syndrome is associated with underdevelopment of the zygomatic bone, down-slanting palpebral fissures, and deformed lower eyelids and external ears.

7–C. The parathyroid and thymus migrate in a caudal and medial direction during development; therefore, ectopic glandular tissue may be found anywhere along the migratory path.

8–H. The inferior parathyroid gland develops from pharyngeal pouch 3.

9–B. The muscles of facial expression develop from pharyngeal arch 2 and are therefore innervated by the facial nerve (CN VII).

10–I. The ultimobranchial body develops from pharyngeal pouch 4.

11–F. The tubotympanic recess forms from pharyngeal pouch 1. The distal portion develops into the middle ear cavity, and the proximal portion develops into the auditory tube.

12–C. Pharyngeal arch 3 is associated with the glossopharyngeal nerve (CN IX).

13–A. The muscles of mastication develop from pharyngeal arch 1 and are therefore innervated by the trigeminal nerve (CN V).

14–A. The maxilla bone of the skull develops from pharyngeal arch 1, specifically from the maxillary prominence.

15–H. The thymus develops from pharyngeal pouch 3.

16–G. The palatine tonsil develops from pharyngeal pouch 2.

17–B. Pharyngeal arch 2 is associated with the facial nerve (CN VII).

18–D. The constrictors of the pharynx develop from pharyngeal arch 4 and are therefore innervated by the superior laryngeal branch of the vagus nerve (CN X).

19–E. The intrinsic muscles of the larynx develop from pharyngeal arch 6 and are therefore innervated by the recurrent laryngeal branch of the vagus nerve (CN X).

13

Urinary System

I. Overview (Figure 13-1)

– The **intermediate mesoderm** forms a longitudinal elevation along the dorsal body wall called the **urogenital ridge**.

– Part of the urogenital ridge forms the **nephrogenic cord**, which gives rise to the urinary system.

– The nephrogenic cord develops into three sets of nephric structures: the **pronephros, mesonephros,** and **metanephros**.

A. The pronephros (Figure 13-2)

– develops by the differentiation of mesoderm within the nephrogenic cord to form **pronephric tubules** and the **pronephric duct**.

– is the cranialmost nephric structure.

– is a transitory structure that regresses completely by week 5 of development and is not functional in humans.

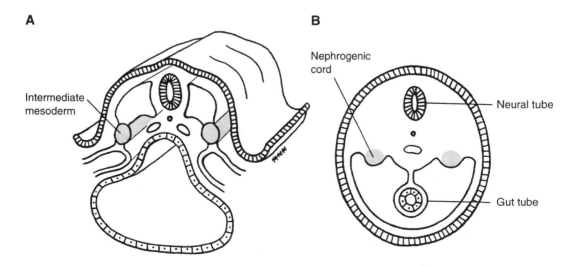

A

B

Intermediate mesoderm

Nephrogenic cord

Neural tube

Gut tube

Figure 13-1. *(A)* Cross-sectional view of an embryo during lateral folding, illustrating the intermediate mesoderm as a cord of mesoderm extending from the cervical to sacral level that forms the urogenital ridge and nephrogenic cord. *(B)* Cross-sectional view of an embryo after lateral folding has occurred, illustrating the nephrogenic cord. (Reprinted from Dudek RW: *High-Yield Embryology.* Baltimore, Williams & Wilkins, 1996, p. 33.)

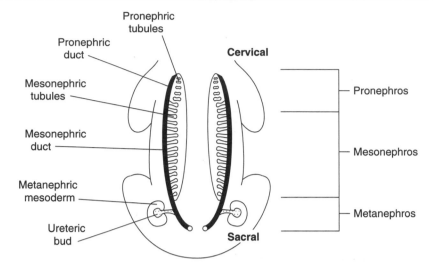

Figure 13-2. Frontal view of an embryo, depicting the pronephros, mesonephros, and metanephros. Note that nephric structures develop from cervical through sacral levels.

B. The mesonephros (see Figure 13-2)

- develops by the differentiation of mesoderm within the nephrogenic cord to form **mesonephric tubules** and the **mesonephric duct (wolffian duct)**.
- is the middle nephric structure.
- is partially transitory and is functional for a short period.
- Most of the mesonephric tubules regress, but the mesonephric duct persists and opens into the urogenital sinus.

C. The metanephros (see Figure 13-2)

- develops from an outgrowth of the mesonephric duct, the **ureteric bud**, and from a condensation of mesoderm within the nephrogenic cord, the **metanephric mesoderm**.
- is the caudalmost nephric structure.
- begins to form at week 5 and is functional in the fetus at about week 10 of development.
- develops into the **definitive adult kidney**.

II. Development of the Kidneys

A. Further development of the metanephros (Figure 13-3 and Table 13-1)

- The ureteric bud initially penetrates the metanephric mesoderm and then undergoes repeated divisions to form the **ureters, renal pelvis, major calyces, minor calyces,** and **collecting ducts**.
- The collecting ducts induce the metanephric mesoderm to form **metanephric vesicles,** which are critical to nephron formation.

1. Nephron formation

- The metanephric vesicles differentiate into the **connecting tubule, distal convoluted tubule, loop of Henle, proximal convoluted tubule, Bowman's capsule,** and the **glomerulus,** all of which form the nephron.

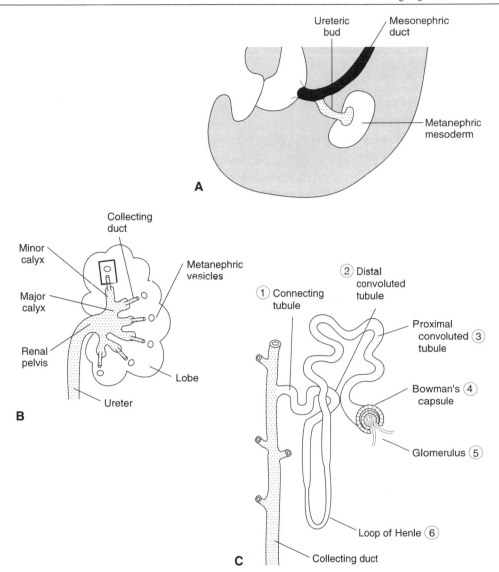

Figure 13-3. *(A)* Lateral view of an embryo showing the ureteric bud *(stippled area)* and the metanephric mesoderm. *(B)* Lateral view of a fetal kidney. *Stippled area* indicates structures formed from the ureteric bud. Note the lobulated appearance of a fetal kidney. The lobulation disappears during infancy as the kidney grows through elongation of the proximal convoluted tubules and loops of Henle. *(C)* Enlarged view of the rectangle shown in *B*, illustrating a collecting duct *(stippled)* derived from the ureteric bud and those structures derived from the metanephric vesicle. Structures numbered 1–6 make up a nephron.

- Nephron formation is complete at birth, but functional maturation of nephrons continues throughout infancy.
- The fetal kidney is divided into **lobes** in contrast to the definitive adult kidney.

2. Tissue sources

- The **transitional epithelium** lining the ureter, pelvis, major calyx, and minor calyx and the **simple cuboidal epithelium** lining the collecting ducts are derived from **mesoderm of the ureteric bud**.

Table 13-1. Development of the Kidneys

Embryonic Structure	Adult Derivative
Ureteric bud	Collecting duct Minor calyces Major calyces Renal pelvis Ureter
Metanephric mesoderm	Renal glomerulus (capillaries) Renal (Bowman's) capsule Proximal convoluted tubule Loop of Henle Distal convoluted tubule Connecting tubule

(Modified from Dudek RW: *High-Yield Embryology.* Baltimore, Williams & Wilkins, 1996, p. 34)

- The **simple cuboidal epithelium** lining the connecting tubule and distal convoluted tubule, the **simple squamous epithelium** lining the loop of Henle, the **simple columnar epithelium** lining the proximal convoluted tubule, and the **podocytes and simple squamous epithelium** lining Bowman's capsule are derived from **mesoderm of the metanephric vesicle**.

B. Relative ascent of the kidneys

- The fetal metanephros is located in the sacral region, whereas the definitive adult kidney is located at **vertebral levels T12–L3**.
- The change in location results from a disproportionate growth of the embryo caudal to the metanephros.
- During the relative ascent, the kidneys rotate 90° medially, causing the hilum to orientate medially.

C. Blood supply of the kidneys

- changes as the metanephros undergoes its relative ascent.
- The metanephros will receive its blood supply from arteries at progressively higher levels until the definitive **renal arteries** develop at L2.
- Arteries formed during the ascent may persist and are called **supernumerary arteries**.
- Supernumerary arteries are **end arteries**; therefore, any damage to them will result in necrosis of kidney parenchyma.

III. Development of the Urinary Bladder (Figure 13-4)

- The urinary bladder is formed from the upper end of the urogenital sinus, which is continuous with the allantois.
- The allantois becomes a fibrous cord, the **urachus (median umbilical ligament)** in the adult.
- The lower ends of the mesonephric ducts become incorporated into the posterior wall of the bladder at the **trigone**.
- The mesonephric ducts eventually open into the urogenital sinus below the bladder.
- The **transitional epithelium** lining the urinary bladder is derived from endoderm because of its etiology from the urogenital sinus and gut tube. The **transi-**

A

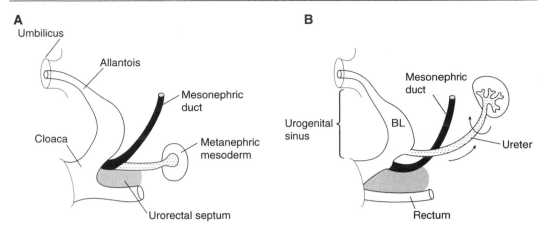

Figure 13-4. Lateral views depicting the formation of the bladder from the upper part of the urogenital sinus at week 4 *(A)* and week 7 *(B)*. Note that the mesonephric duct *(black)* and ureteric bud *(stippled)* undergo separation and obtain their own opening. The urorectal septum *(shaded)* partitions the cloaca to form the rectum (hindgut) and urogenital sinus. *Arrows* indicate the relative ascent and medial rotation of the kidneys. *BL* = bladder.

tional epithelium lining the ureters, renal pelvis, and major and minor calyces is derived from mesoderm because of its etiology from the ureteric bud.

IV. Development of the Female Urethra (Figure 13-5)

– The female urethra is formed from the lower end of the urogenital sinus.
– develops endodermal outgrowths into the surrounding mesoderm to form the **urethral glands** and **paraurethral glands**.
– ends at the **vestibule of the vagina**, which also forms from the urogenital sinus. The vestibule of the vagina develops endodermal outgrowths into the surrounding mesoderm to form the **greater vestibular glands**.
– The **transitional epithelium** and **stratified squamous epithelium** lining the female urethra are derived from **endoderm**.

V. Development of the Male Urethra (Figure 13-6)

A. Prostatic urethra, membranous urethra, and proximal part of penile urethra

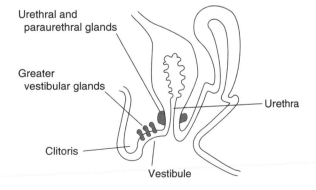

Figure 13-5. Diagram depicting the female urethra.

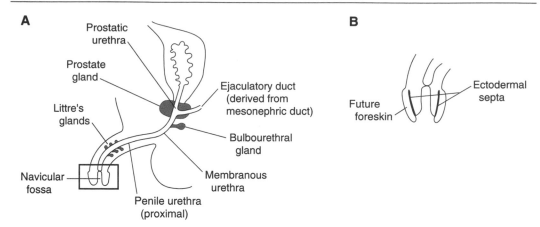

Figure 13-6. *(A)* Diagram depicting the male urethra. Note that the ejaculatory duct, which is derived from the mesonephric duct, opens into the prostatic urethra. *(B)* Enlarged view of box in *A*, showing the formation of the foreskin.

- These parts of the urethra are formed from the lower end of the urogenital sinus.
- The **transitional epithelium** and **stratified columnar epithelium** lining these parts of the urethra are derived from **endoderm**.

1. The **prostatic urethra** develops endodermal outgrowths into the surrounding mesoderm to form the **prostate gland**.

2. The **membranous urethra** develops endodermal outgrowths into the surrounding mesoderm to form the **bulbourethral glands**.

3. The **proximal part of the penile urethra** develops endodermal outgrowths into the surrounding mesoderm to form **Littre's glands**.

B. **Distal part of the penile urethra**

- is formed from an ingrowth of surface ectoderm called the **glandular plate**.
- The glandular plate joins the penile urethra and becomes canalized to form the **navicular fossa**.
- Ectodermal septa appear lateral to the navicular fossa and become canalized to form the **foreskin**.
- The **stratified squamous epithelium** lining this part of the urethra is derived from **ectoderm**.

VI. Development of the Suprarenal Gland

A. **Cortex**

- forms from **two episodes of mesoderm proliferation** between the root of the dorsal mesentery and the gonad; the first episode forms the primitive **fetal cortex**, and the second forms the definitive **adult cortex**.
- The fetal cortex is present at birth but regresses by the second postnatal month.
- The zona glomerulosa and zona fasciculata of the definitive cortex are also present at birth, but the zona reticularis is not formed until age 3 years.

B. Medulla

- forms when **neural crest cells** aggregate at the medial aspect of the fetal cortex and eventually become surrounded by the fetal cortex.
- The neural crest cells differentiate into **epinephrine** and **norepinephrine-containing cells**, which stain yellow-brown with chromium salts and hence are called **chromaffin cells**.
- Chromaffin cells can be found in extrasuprarenal sites at birth, but these sites normally will regress completely by puberty: In a normal adult, chromaffin cells are found only in the suprarenal medulla.

VII. Clinical Considerations

A. Renal agenesis

- occurs when the **ureteric bud fails to develop**, thereby eliminating the induction of metanephric vesicles and nephron formation.

1. Unilateral renal agenesis

- is relatively common; therefore, a physician should never assume a patient has two kidneys.
- is more common in males.
- is asymptomatic and compatible with life because the remaining kidney hypertrophies.

2. Bilateral renal agenesis

- is relatively uncommon.
- causes oligohydramnios during pregnancy, which allows the uterine wall to compress the fetus, resulting in **Potter syndrome** (deformed limbs, wrinkly skin, and abnormal facial appearance).
- is incompatible with life unless a suitable donor is available for kidney transplant.

B. Pelvic kidney

- is an ectopic kidney that occurs when one or both kidneys fail to ascend and therefore remain in the pelvis or lower lumbar area.
- In some cases, two pelvic kidneys fuse to form a solid mass, commonly called a **pancake kidney**.

C. Horseshoe kidney

- occurs when the inferior poles of the kidneys fuse.
- Normal ascent of the kidneys is arrested because the fused portion gets trapped behind the **inferior mesenteric artery**.

D. Duplication of the urinary tract

- occurs when the ureteric bud prematurely divides before penetrating the metanephric mesoderm.
- results in either a double kidney or duplicated ureter and renal pelvis.

E. Polycystic disease of the kidneys

- occurs when the loops of Henle dilate, forming large cysts that severely compromise kidney function.
- is a relatively common hereditary disease.
- is associated clinically with cysts of the liver, pancreas, and lungs.

– Treatment includes dialysis and kidney transplant.

F. Exstrophy of the bladder

– occurs when the posterior wall of the urinary bladder is exposed to the exterior.
– is caused by a failure of the anterior abdominal wall and anterior wall of the bladder to develop properly.
– is associated clinically with urine drainage to the exterior and **epispadias**.
– Surgical reconstruction is difficult and prolonged.

G. Urachal cyst or sinus

– occurs when a remnant of the allantois persists, thereby forming a cyst or sinus.
– is found along the midline on a path from the umbilicus to the apex of the urinary bladder.
– is often associated clinically with urine drainage from the umbilicus.

H. Ectopic ureteric orifices

– In males, the ectopic ureter usually opens into the neck of the bladder or prostatic urethra.
– In females, the ectopic ureter usually opens into the neck of the bladder or vestibule of the vagina.
– Incontinence is the common complaint since urine continually dribbles from the urethra in males and the urethra or vagina in females.

I. Pheochromocytoma

– is a relatively rare chromaffin cell neoplasm containing epinephrine and nor-epinephrine
– occurs mainly in adults 40–60 years old.
– is generally found in the region of the suprarenal gland, but may be found in extrasuprarenal sites.
– is clinically associated with **persistent or paroxysmal hypertension** due to epinephrine secretion, which can be cured by surgical excision of the neoplasm.

J. Neuroblastoma

– is a very common extracranial neoplasm containing primitive neuroblasts of neural crest origin.
– occurs mainly in children.
– 60% of neuroblastomas are found in extrasuprarenal sites generally along the sympathetic chain ganglia; the remaining 40% are found within the adrenal medulla.

K. Wilms' tumor

– is the most common renal tumor of childhood; usually diagnosed between 2 and 5 years of age.
– the tumor tends to be a large, solitary, well- circumscribed mass that is tan to gray in color.
– the histological appearance resembles a recapitulation of embryological formation with three classic areas described: (1) a stromal area, (2) tightly-packed embryonic cells, and (3) small tubules.

Review Test

Directions: Each of the numbered items or incomplete statements in this section is followed by answers or by completions of the statement. Select the **one** lettered answer or completion that is **best** in each case.

1. When does the metanephros become functional?

(A) at week 3 of development
(B) at week 4 of development
(C) at week 10 of development
(D) just before birth
(E) just after birth

2. A urachal cyst is a remnant of the

(A) urogenital sinus
(B) urogenital ridge
(C) cloaca
(D) allantois
(E) mesonephric duct

3. During surgery for a benign cyst on the kidney, the surgeon notes that the patient's right kidney has two ureters and two renal pelves. This malformation is

(A) an abnormal division of the pronephros
(B) an abnormal division of the mesonephros
(C) formation of an extra mass of intermediate mesoderm
(D) a premature division of the metanephric mesoderm
(E) a premature division of the ureteric bud

4. The transitional epithelium lining the urinary bladder is derived from

(A) ectoderm
(B) endoderm
(C) mesoderm
(D) endoderm and mesoderm
(E) neural crest cells

5. The transitional epithelium lining the ureter is derived from

(A) ectoderm
(B) endoderm
(C) mesoderm
(D) endoderm and mesoderm
(E) neural crest cells

6. The podocytes of Bowman's capsule are derived from

(A) ectoderm
(B) endoderm
(C) mesoderm
(D) endoderm and mesoderm
(E) neural crest cells

7. The proximal convoluted tubules of the definitive adult kidney are derived from the

(A) ureteric bud
(B) metanephric vesicle
(C) mesonephric duct
(D) mesonephric tubules
(E) pronephric tubules

8. The trigone on the posterior wall of the urinary bladder is formed by the

(A) incorporation of the lower end of the mesonephric ducts
(B) incorporation of the lower end of the pronephric ducts
(C) incorporation of the metanephric mesoderm
(D) incorporation of the mesonephric tubules
(E) incorporation of the pronephric tubules

9. A 6-year-old girl presents with a large abdominal mass just superior to the pubic symphysis. The mass is tender when palpated and fixed in location. During surgery, a fluid-filled mass is noted connected to the umbilicus superiorly and to the urinary bladder inferiorly. What is the diagnosis?

(A) pelvic kidney
(B) horseshoe kidney
(C) polycystic disease of the kidney
(D) urachal cyst
(E) exstrophy of the bladder

10. Immediately after birth of a boy, a moist, red protrusion of tissue is noted just superior to his pubic symphysis. After observation, urine drainage is noted from the upper lateral corners of this tissue mass. What is the diagnosis?

(A) pelvic kidney
(B) horseshoe kidney
(C) polycystic disease of the kidney
(D) urachal cyst
(E) exstrophy of the bladder

Directions: Each group of items in this section consists of lettered options followed by a set of numbered items. For each item, select the **one** lettered option that is most closely associated with it. Each lettered option may be selected once, more than once, or not at all.

Questions 11–20

For each of the following characteristics, choose the most appropriate nephric structure.

(A) Pronephros
(B) Mesonephros
(C) Metanephros
(D) Ureteric bud
(E) Metanephric vesicle

11. The caudalmost kidney

12. The cranialmost kidney

13. Completely regresses

14. Forms the ureter

15. Forms the loop of Henle

16. Forms Bowman's capsule

17. Forms the collecting ducts

18. The kidney that is functional at birth

19. Develops from an outgrowth of the meso-nephric duct

20. Is formed by the inductive influence of the collecting ducts

Answers and Explanations

1–C. The metanephros begins to form at week 5 and starts to function in the fetus at about week 10. The pronephros is not functional in humans. The mesonephros is the interim kidney, which functions until the metanephros is ready.

2–D. The upper end of the urogenital sinus is in patent communication with the allantois, which lies in the umbilical cord. The allantois normally regresses and forms a fibrous cord. If a remnant persists, it forms a urachal cyst or sinus.

3–E. The ureteric bud seems to be preprogrammed to undergo repeated divisions. These divisions normally begin on contact with the metanephric mesoderm. If the ureteric bud undergoes division prematurely, duplication of the ureter and renal pelvis occurs. In some circumstances, two separate kidneys may form.

4–B. The transitional epithelium lining the urinary bladder is derived from endoderm because the urinary bladder develops from the upper end of the urogenital sinus. The origin of the urogenital sinus can be traced back to the gut tube, which is lined by endoderm.

5–C. The transitional epithelium lining the ureter is derived from mesoderm because the ureter develops from the ureteric bud. The ureteric bud is a diverticulum from the mesonephric duct whose origin can be traced back to the intermediate mesoderm.

6–C. The podocytes of Bowman's capsule develop from the metanephric vesicles, which are of mesodermal origin.

7–B. The connecting tubule, distal convoluted tubule, loop of Henle, proximal convoluted tubule, and Bowman's capsule are all derived from the metanephric vesicle.

8–A. The lower end of the mesonephric ducts are incorporated into the posterior wall of the urinary bladder. The mesonephric ducts contribute to the connective tissue component of the posterior wall at the trigone. It is generally believed that the transitional epithelium lining the entire bladder (even the trigone) is of endodermal origin.

9–D. A urachal cyst or sinus forms from a remnant of the allantois and is found along the midline on a path from the umbilicus to the apex of the urinary bladder. The epithelium lining the cyst produces secretions that gradually fill the remnant with fluid. Very rarely, the entire allantois persists, forming a fistula that is patent from the urinary bladder to the exterior at the umbilicus.

10–E. The moist, red tissue mass that is exposed to the exterior is actually the posterior wall of the urinary bladder. This is called exstrophy of the bladder and is caused when the anterior abdominal wall and anterior wall of the bladder fail to form. The ureters open onto the posterior wall; therefore, urine drainage is apparent.

11–C. The nephrogenic cord extends along the entire dorsal body wall and develops into the pronephros, mesonephros, and metanephros. The metanephros, the caudalmost kidney, develops in the sacral region.

12–A. The nephrogenic cord extends along the entire dorsal body wall and develops into the pronephros, mesonephros, and metanephros. The pronephros, the cranialmost kidney, develops in the cervical region.

13–A. The pronephros completely regresses by week 5 of development and is never functional in the human. For this reason, many authorities believe that the concept of the pronephros does not apply to humans.

14–D. The ureteric bud forms the ureter.

15–E. The metanephric vesicle forms the loop of Henle.

16–E. The metanephric vesicle forms Bowman's capsule.

17–D. The ureteric bud penetrates the metanephric mesoderm and undergoes repeated divisions to form the collecting ducts.

18–C. The metanephros begins to form at week 5 of embryonic development and is functional at about week 10. At birth, the metanephros (definitive kidney) is functional.

19–D. The ureteric bud develops as an outgrowth of the mesonephric duct.

20–E. The collecting ducts induce the formation of the metanephric vesicles, which are critical to nephron development.

14

Female Reproductive System

I. The Indifferent Embryo

– Although the genotype of the embryo (46,XX or 46,XY) is established at fertilization, the embryo during weeks 1–6 remains in a sexually **indifferent** or **undifferentiated stage**; that is, genetically female embryos and genetically male embryos are phenotypically indistinguishable.

– The indifferent embryo begins phenotypic sexual differentiation during week 7 of development; by week 12 female or male characteristics of the external genitalia can be recognized; by about week 20 phenotypic differentiation is complete.

– Phenotypic sexual differentiation may result in individuals with a **female** phenotype, an **intersex** phenotype, or a **male** phenotype.

– The components of the indifferent embryo that are remodeled to form the adult female reproductive system are the **gonads, genital ducts,** and **primordia of the external genitalia**. Phenotypic sexual differentiation occurs in a sequence beginning with the gonads, then the genital ducts, and finally with the primordia of the external genitalia.

A. The gonads

– The indifferent embryo has one pair of gonads that develop into either the ovaries or testes.

B. Genital ducts

– The indifferent embryo has two types of genital ducts.

1. **Paramesonephric (müllerian) ducts** play a major role in the female.

2. **Mesonephric (wolffian) ducts** and **tubules** play a major role in the male.

C. Primordia of external genitalia

1. **Phallus**

2. **Urethral folds**

3. **Genital swellings**

II. Development of the Gonads (Figure 14-1)

A. The Ovary

– The **intermediate mesoderm** forms a longitudinal elevation along the dorsal body wall, the **urogenital ridge**.

– The coelomic epithelium and underlying mesoderm of the urogenital ridge proliferate to form the **gonadal ridge**.

– **Primary sex cords** develop from the gonadal ridge and incorporate **primordial germ cells (XX genotype)**, which migrate into the gonad from the wall of the yolk sac.

– Primary sex cords develop into the **rete ovarii**, which degenerate.

– Later, **secondary sex cords** develop and incorporate primordial germ cells as a thin **tunica albuginea** forms.

– The secondary sex cords break apart and form isolated cell clusters called **primordial follicles**, which contain **primary oocytes** surrounded by a layer of **simple squamous cells**.

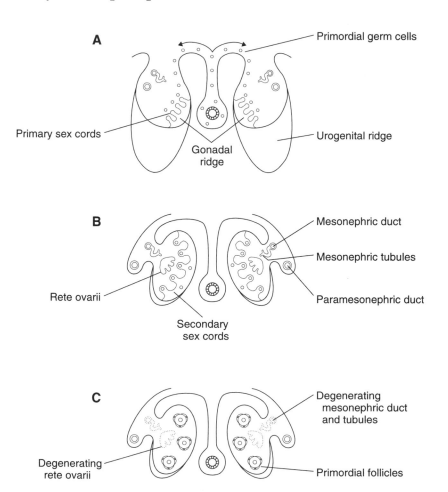

Figure 14-1. Diagram indicating the differentiation of the gonad in the female. *(A)* Gonad in the indifferent embryo. *(B)* Ovary at week 12 of development. *(C)* Ovary at week 20.

- Primary oocytes, simple squamous cells, and connective tissue stroma of the ovary are derived from mesoderm.

B. Relative descent of the ovaries

- The ovaries originally develop within the abdomen but later undergo a relative descent into the pelvis as a result of disproportionate growth of the upper abdominal region away from the pelvic region.
- Other factors in this movement are uncertain but probably include the **gubernaculum**, a band of fibrous tissue along the posterior wall that extends from the medial pole of the ovary to the uterus at the junction of the uterine tubes, forming the **ovarian ligament**, and then continues into the labia majora, forming the **round ligament of the uterus.**
- The peritoneum evaginates alongside the gubernaculum to form the **processus vaginalis**, which is obliterated in the female later in development.

III. Development of Genital Ducts (Figure 14-2)

A. Paramesonephric ducts

- develop as invaginations of the lateral surface of the urogenital ridge.
- The cranial portions develop into the uterine tubes.
- The caudal portions fuse in the midline to form the **uterovaginal primordium** and thereby bring together two peritoneal folds called the **broad ligament.**
- The **uterovaginal primordium** develops into the **uterus, cervix,** and **superior one-third of the vagina**.
- The paramesonephric ducts project into the dorsal wall of the urogenital sinus and induce the formation of the **sinovaginal bulbs**.
- The sinovaginal bulbs fuse to form the solid **vaginal plate**, which canalizes and develops into the **inferior two-thirds of the vagina.**
- Although the vagina has a dual origin, most authorities agree that the epithelial lining of the entire vagina is of **endodermal origin.**
- Vestigial remnants of the paramesonephric duct may be found in the adult female and are called the **hydatid of Morgagni.**

B. Mesonephric ducts and tubules

- develop in the female as part of the urinary system since these ducts are critical in the formation of the definitive metanephric kidney. However, they regress in the female after formation of the metanephric kidney.
- Vestigial remnants of the mesonephric ducts called the **appendix vesiculosa** and **Gartner's duct** may be found in the adult female.
- Vestigial remnants of the mesonephric tubules called the **epoöphoron** and **paroöphoron** may be found in the adult female.

IV. Development of the Primordia of the External Genitalia (Figure 14-3)

- A proliferation of mesoderm around the cloacal membrane causes the overlying ectoderm to rise up so that three structures are visible externally: the **phallus, urethral folds,** and **genital swellings**.
- The phallus forms the **clitoris.**
- The urethral folds form the **labia minora.**

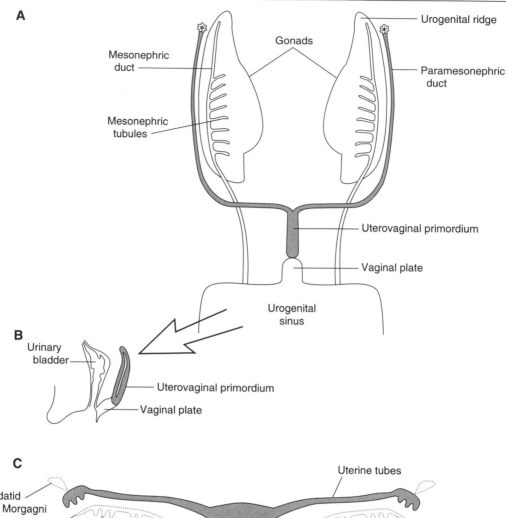

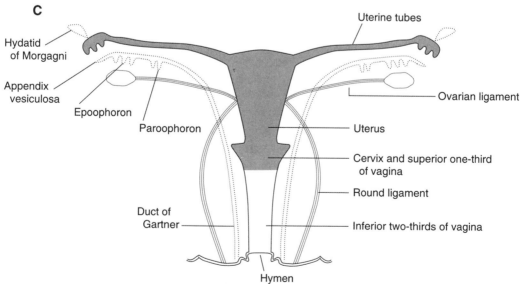

Figure 14-2. Diagram indicating the differentiation of the genital ducts in the female. *(A)* Genital ducts in the indifferent embryo. *(B)* Side view showing the dual origin of the vagina. *(C)* Female components and vestigial remnants *(dotted lines)* at birth. The paramesonephric ducts and their derivatives are *shaded.*

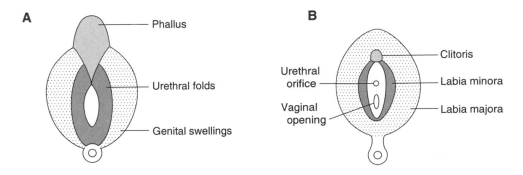

Figure 14-3. Diagram indicating the differentiation of the phallus, urethral folds, and genital swellings in the female. *(A)* Primordia at week 5 of development. *(B)* Female external genitalia at birth.

– The genital swellings form the **labia majora** and **mons pubis**.

V. Clinical Considerations (Figure 14-4)

A. Double uterus with double vagina
– is a condition where two uteri and two vaginas are present.
– results from the complete lack of fusion of the paramesonephric ducts and the sinovaginal bulbs.

B. Bicornuate uterus
– is a condition in which the uterus has two horns entering a common vagina.
– results from partial fusion of the paramesonephric ducts.

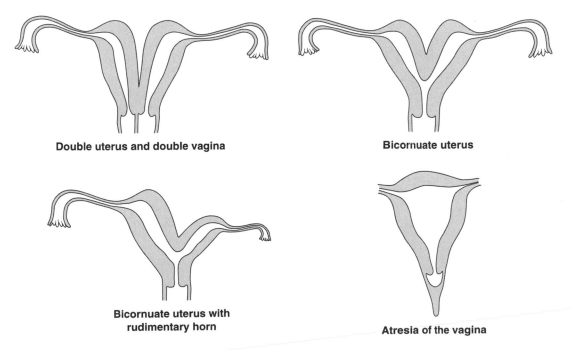

Figure 14-4. Diagram depicting various congenital anomalies of the uterus and vagina.

C. Bicornuate uterus with rudimentary horn
– is a condition in which only one side of the uterus forms normally.
– results from retarded growth of one of the paramesonephric ducts.

D. Absence of uterus and vagina
– is a condition where no uterus or vagina is present.
– results from the failure of the paramesonephric ducts and the sinovaginal bulbs to develop.

E. Atresia of the vagina
– is a condition where the vaginal lumen is blocked.
– results from failure of the vaginal plate to canalize and form a lumen.
– When only the inferior part of the vaginal plate fails to canalize, a condition known as imperforate hymen occurs.

VI. Summary of Female Reproductive System Development (see Table 15-1)

Review Test

Directions: Each of the numbered items or incomplete statements in this section is followed by answers or by completions of the statement. Select the **one** lettered answer or completion that is **best** in each case.

1. The indifferent embryo begins phenotypic sexual differentiation during

(A) week 3 of development
(B) week 5 of development
(C) week 7 of development
(D) week 12 of development
(E) week 20 of development

2. The indifferent embryo completes phenotypic sexual differentiation during

(A) week 3 of development
(B) week 5 of development
(C) week 7 of development
(D) week 12 of development
(E) week 20 of development

3. After the sinovaginal bulbs have proliferated and fused, they form a solid core of endodermal cells called the:

(A) vestibule of the vagina
(B) uterovaginal primordium
(C) urogenital sinus
(D) vaginal plate
(E) clitoris

4. A structure found within the adult female pelvis formed from the gubernaculum is the

(A) broad ligament
(B) suspensory ligament of the ovary
(C) round ligament of the uterus
(D) medial umbilical ligament
(E) median umbilical ligament

5. The labia minora arise embryologically from which of the following structures?

(A) phallus
(B) genital swellings
(C) sinovaginal bulbs
(D) urethral folds
(E) paramesonephric duct

6. The uterine tubes of the adult female are derived embryologically from which of the following?

(A) mesonephric duct
(B) mesonephric tubules
(C) paramesonephric duct
(D) paramesonephric tubules
(E) uterovaginal primordium

Directions: Each group of items in this section consists of lettered options followed by a set of numbered items. For each item, select the **one** lettered option that is most closely associated with it. Each lettered option may be selected once, more than once, or not at all.

Questions 7-14

For each of the adult structures below, choose the most appropriate embryonic structure from which it is derived.

(A) Paramesonephic duct
(B) Mesonephric duct
(C) Mesonephric tubules
(D) Phallus
(E) Urethral folds
(F) Genital swellings

7. Uterus

8. Clitoris

9. Labia minora

10. Gartner's duct

11. Cervix

12. Labia majora

13. Hydatid of Morgagni

14. Epoöphoron

Answers and Explanations

1–C. The embryo during weeks 1–6 remains in an indifferent or undifferentiated stage. The embryo begins phenotypic sexual differentiation during week 7.

2–E. By week 12, female and male characteristics can be recognized. By week 20, phenotypic sexual differentiation is complete.

3–D. The sinovaginal bulbs proliferate, fuse, and form the vaginal plate under the inductive influence of the paramesonephric ducts. The vaginal plate then canalizes to form the inferior two-thirds of the vagina.

4–C. The round ligament of the uterus and the ovarian ligament both form from the gubernaculum.

5–D. In the female, the urethral folds remain unfused and form the labia minora.

6–C. The cranial portion of the paramesonephric ducts form the uterine tubes.

7–A. The uterus forms from the paramesonephric duct.

8–D. The clitoris forms from the phallus.

9–E. The labia minora form from the urethral folds.

10–B. Gartner's duct is a remnant of the mesonephric duct in the female.

11–A. The cervix, which is part of the uterus, forms from the paramesonephric duct.

12–F. The labia majora form from the genital swellings.

13–A. Although the paramesonephric ducts form many important structures in the female, a vestigial remnant of these embryonic ducts may remain and is described as the hydatid of Morgagni.

14–C. The epoöphoron and paroöphoron are remnants of the mesonephric tubules in the female.

15

Male Reproductive System

I. The Indifferent Embryo

– Although the genotype of the embryo (46,XX or 46,XY) is established at fertilization, the embryo during weeks 1–6 remains in a sexually **indifferent** or **undifferentiated stage**; that is, genetically female embryos and genetically male embryos are phenotypically indistinguishable.

– The indifferent embryo begins phenotypic sexual differentiation during week 7 of development; by week 12 female or male characteristics of the external genitalia can be recognized; by about week 20 phenotypic differentiation is complete.

– Phenotypic sexual differentiation may result in individuals with a **female** phenotype, an **intersex** phenotype, or a **male** phenotype.

– The components of the indifferent embryo that are remodeled to form the adult female reproductive system are the **gonads, genital ducts,** and **primordia of the external genitalia**. Phenotypic sexual differentiation occurs in a sequence beginning with the gonads, then the genital ducts, and finally with the primordia of the external genitalia.

A. The gonads

– The indifferent embryo has one pair of gonads that develop into either the ovaries or testes.

B. Genital ducts

– The indifferent embryo has two types of genital ducts.

1. **Paramesonephric (müllerian) ducts** play a major role in the female.

2. **Mesonephric (wolffian) ducts** and **tubules** play a major role in the male.

C. Primordia of external genitalia

1. **Phallus**

2. **Urethral folds**

3. **Genital swellings**

II. Development of the Gonads (Figure 15-1)

A. The Testes

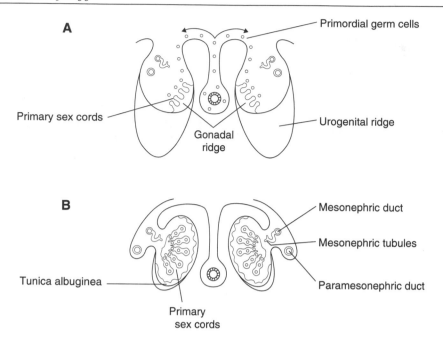

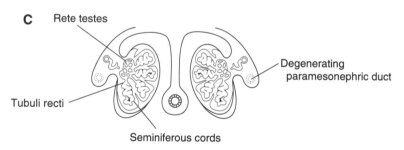

Figure 15-1. Diagram indicating the differentiation of the gonad in the male. *(A)* Gonad in the indifferent embryo. *(B)* Testes at week 7 of development. *(C)* Testes at week 20.

- The **intermediate mesoderm** forms a longitudinal elevation along the dorsal body wall, the **urogenital ridge.**
- The coelomic epithelium and underlying mesoderm of the urogenital ridge proliferate to form the **gonadal ridge.**
- **Primary sex cords** develop from the gonadal ridge and incorporate **primordial germ cells (XY genotype),** which migrate into the gonad from the wall of the yolk sac.
- The Y chromosome carries a gene on its short arm that codes for **testes-determining factor (TDF),** which is crucial to testes differentiation.
- The primary sex cords extend into the medulla of the gonad and lose their connection with the surface epithelium as the thick **tunica albuginea** forms.
- The primary sex cords form the **seminiferous cords, tubuli recti,** and **rete testes.**
- Seminiferous cords consist of **primordial germ cells** and **sustentacular (Sertoli) cells,** which secrete **müllerian-inhibiting factor (MIF).**

- The mesoderm between the seminiferous cords gives rise to the **interstitial (Leydig) cells**, which secrete **testosterone**.
- The primordial germ cells, sustentacular (Sertoli) cells, interstitial (Leydig) cells, and connective tissue stroma of the testes are derived from mesoderm.
- The seminiferous cords remain as solid cords until puberty, when they acquire a lumen and are then called **seminiferous tubules**.

B. Relative descent of the testes

- The testes originally develop within the abdomen but later descend into the scrotum. The relative descent of the testes to the inguinal canal is a result of disproportionate growth of the upper abdominal region away from the pelvic region.
- Factors involved in the final descent of the testes into the scrotum are uncertain; however, it seems that increased pressure due to the **growth of abdominal viscera**, the **gubernaculum**, and **testosterone** is involved.
- The gubernaculum in the male is a band of fibrous tissue along the posterior wall that extends from the caudal pole of the testes to the scrotum. Remnants of the gubernaculum in the adult male serve to anchor the testes within the scrotum.
- The peritoneum evaginates alongside the gubernaculum to form the **processus vaginalis**. Later in development, most of the processus vaginalis is obliterated except at its distal end, which remains as a peritoneal sac called the **tunica vaginalis** of the testes.

III. Development of Genital Ducts (Figure 15-2)

A. Paramesonephric ducts

- develop as invaginations of the lateral surface of the urogenital ridge.
- The cranial portions run parallel to the mesonephric ducts.
- The caudal portions fuse in the midline to form the **uterovaginal primordium**.
- Under the influence of MIF, the cranial portions of the paramesonephric ducts and the uterovaginal primordium regress completely.
- Vestigial remnants of the paramesonephric duct called the **appendix testis** may be found in the adult male.

B. Mesonephric ducts and tubules

- develop in the male as part of the urinary system since these ducts are critical in the formation of the definitive metanephric kidney.
- The **mesonephric ducts** then proceed to additionally form the **epididymis, ductus deferens, seminal vesicle,** and **ejaculatory duct**.
- A few **mesonephric tubules** in the region of the testes form the **efferent ductules** of the testes.
- Vestigial remnants of the mesonephric duct called the **appendix epididymis** may be found in the adult male.
- Vestigial remnants of mesonephric tubules called the **paradidymis** may be found in the adult male.

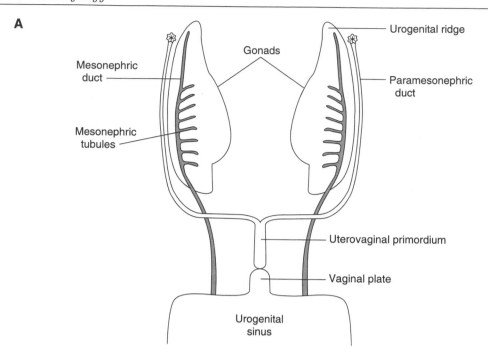

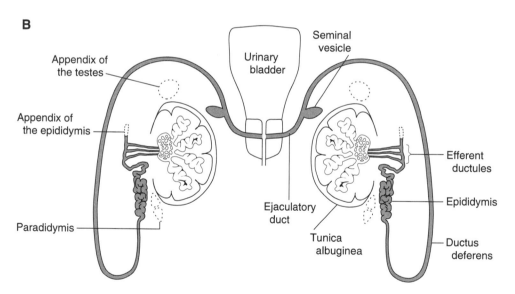

Figure 15-2. Diagram indicating the differentiation of the genital ducts in the male. *(A)* Genital ducts in the indifferent embryo. *(B)* Male components and vestigial remnants *(dotted lines)*. The mesonephric ducts/tubules and their derivatives are *shaded*.

IV. Development of the Primordia of the External Genitalia
(Figure 15-3)

– A proliferation of mesoderm around the cloacal membrane causes the overlying ectoderm to rise up so that three structures are visible externally: the **phallus**, **urethral folds**, and **genital swellings**.

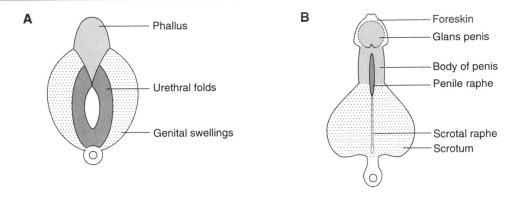

Figure 15-3. Diagram indicating the differentiation of the phallus, urethral folds, and genital swellings in the male. *(A)* Primordium at week 5 of development. *(B)* Male external genitalia at birth.

- The phallus forms **glans** and **body of the penis**.
- The urethral folds form the **penile raphe**.
- The genital swellings form the **scrotum** and **scrotal raphe**.

V. Clinical Considerations

A. Intersexuality

- Because the early embryo goes through an indifferent stage, events may occur whereby a fetus does not progress toward either of the two usual phenotypes but gets caught in an intermediate stage known as intersexuality.
- is classified according to the **histologic appearance of the gonad** and **ambiguous genitalia**.

1. True intersexuality

- occurs when an individual has both ovarian and testicular tissue (**ovotestes**) histologically and ambiguous genitalia.
- Individuals usually have a 46,XX genotype.
- is a rare condition whose cause is poorly understood.

2. Female pseudointersexuality

- occurs when an individual has only ovarian tissue histologically and masculinization of the female external genitalia.
- Individuals have a 46,XX genotype.
- Most common cause is **congenital adrenal hyperplasia**, a condition in which the fetus produces excess androgens.

3. Male pseudointersexuality

- occurs when an individual has only testicular tissue histologically and various stages of stunted development of the male external genitalia.
- Individuals have a 46,XY genotype.
- Most common cause is inadequate production of testosterone and MIF by the fetal testes.

B. Gonadal dysgenesis

- occurs when primordial germ cells migrate into the indifferent gonad but later **degenerate**.
- is generally found in individuals with a 45,XO genotype (Turner syndrome).

C. Complete androgen insensitivity (CAIS, or testicular feminization syndrome)

– occurs when a fetus with a 46,XY genotype develops testes and female external genitalia with a rudimentary vagina; uterus and uterine tubes are generally absent.

– Testes may be found in the labia majora and are surgically removed to circumvent malignant tumor formation.

– These individuals present as normal-appearing females, and their psychosocial orientation is female despite their genotype.

– Most common cause is lack of androgen receptors in the urethral folds and genital swellings.

D. Hypospadias

– occurs when the urethral folds fail to fuse completely, resulting in the external urethral orifice opening onto the ventral surface of the penis.

– is generally associated with a poorly developed penis that curves ventrally, known as **chordee**.

E. Epispadias

– occurs when the external urethral orifice opens onto the dorsal surface of the penis.

– is generally associated with exstrophy of the bladder.

F. Undescended testes (cryptorchidism)

– occurs when the testes fail to descend into the scrotum. This normally occurs within 3 months after birth.

– Bilateral cryptorchidism results in sterility.

– The undescended testes may be found in the abdominal cavity or in the inguinal canal.

G. Congenital inguinal hernia

– occurs when a large patency of the processus vaginalis remains so that a loop of intestine may herniate into the scrotum or labia majora.

– is most common in males.

– is generally associated with cryptorchidism.

H. Hydrocele of the testes

– occurs when a small patency of the processus vaginalis remains so that peritoneal fluid can flow into the processus vaginalis.

– results in a fluid-filled cyst near the testes.

VI. Summary of Male Reproductive System Development
(Table 15-1)

Table 15-1. Development of the Male and Female Reproductive Systems

Indifferent Embryo	Adult Female	Adult Male
Gonads	Ovary, primordial follicles, rete ovarii	Testes, seminiferous tubules, tubuli recti rete testes, Leydig cells
Paramesonephric ducts	Uterine tubes, uterus, cervix and superior 1/3 of vagina *Hydatid of Morgagni**	*Appendix testes*
Mesonephric ducts	*Appendix vesiculosa, Gartner's duct*	Epididymis, ductus deferens, seminal vesicles, ejaculatory duct *Appendix epididymis*
Mesonephric tubules	*Epoöphoron, paroöphoron*	Efferent ductules *Paradidymis*
Phallus	Clitoris	Glans and body of penis
Urogenital folds	Labia minora	Penile raphe
Labioscrotal swellings	Labia majora, mons pubis	Scrotum, scrotal raphe
Gubernaculum	Ovarian ligament Round ligament of uterus	Gubernaculum testes
Processus vaginalis	—	Tunica vaginalis

* Italics indicate vestigial structures.

Review Test

Directions: Each of the numbered items or incomplete statements in this section is followed by answers or by completions of the statement. Select the **one** lettered answer or completion that is **best** in each case.

1. Each of the following is characteristic of testicular feminization syndrome EXCEPT

(A) a female phenotype
(B) lack of a uterus
(C) ovaries
(D) 46,XY genotype
(E) testes

2. The most common cause of female pseudointersexuality is

(A) a 46,XO genotype
(B) a 47,XXY genotype
(C) lack of androgen receptors
(D) congenital adrenal hyperplasia
(E) inadequate production of testosterone and müllerian-inhibiting factor (MIF)

3. The most common cause of male pseudointersexuality is

(A) a 45,XO genotype
(B) a 47,XXY genotype
(C) inadequate production of testosterone and müllerian-inhibiting factor (MIF)
(D) congenital adrenal hyperplasia
(E) lack of androgen receptors

4. The most common cause of testicular feminization syndrome is

(A) a 45,XO genotype
(B) a 47,XXY genotype
(C) inadequate production of testosterone and müllerian-inhibiting factor (MIF)
(D) congenital adrenal hyperplasia
(E) lack of androgen receptors

5. In the male, failure of the urethral folds to fuse completely results in

(A) hypospadias
(B) epispadias
(C) cryptorchidism
(D) congenital inguinal hernia
(E) hydrocele

6. The Y chromosome carries a gene on its short arm that codes for

(A) testosterone
(B) müllerian-inhibiting factor (MIF)
(C) testes-determining factor (TDF)
(D) progesterone
(E) estrogen

7. Bilateral cryptorchidism usually results in

(A) impotence
(B) sterility
(C) male pseudointersexuality
(D) female pseudointersexuality
(E) testicular feminization syndrome

8. A 17-year-old girl presents with a complaint of amenorrhea. Physical examination reveals good breast development and normal amount of pubic hair. A rudimentary vagina and a mobile mass within both the right and left labia majora are found on pelvic examination. Ultrasound reveals the absence of a uterus. What is the diagnosis?

(A) testicular feminization syndrome
(B) gonadal dysgenesis
(C) cryptorchidism
(D) female pseudointersexuality
(E) hypospadias

Directions: Each group of items in this section consists of lettered options followed by a set of numbered items. For each item, select the **one** lettered option that is most closely associated with it. Each lettered option may be selected once, more than once, or not at all.

Questions 9–17

For each of the adult structures below, choose the most appropriate embryonic structure from which it is derived.

(A) Paramesonephric duct
(B) Mesonephric duct
(C) Mesonephric tubules
(D) Phallus
(E) Urethral folds
(F) Genital swellings

9. Appendix testis

10. Efferent ductules

11. Epididymis

12. Ductus deferens

13. Glans penis

14. Scrotum

15. Seminal vesicle

16. Penile raphe

17. Ejaculatory duct

Answers and Explanations

1–C. Fetuses with testicular feminization syndrome have a 46,XY genotype, so they develop testes (not ovaries). However, the urethral folds and genital swellings lack androgen receptors so that female genitalia develop. These individuals present as normal-appearing females but lack a uterus because the fetal testes produce müllerian-inhibiting factor (MIF), which causes the regression of the paramesonephric ducts.

2–D. Female pseudointersex individuals have a 46,XX genotype. This condition is most commonly caused by congenital adrenal hyperplasia, in which the fetus produces excessive amounts of androgens. The high androgen level will masculinize the female genitalia.

3–C. Male pseudointersex individuals have a 46,XY genotype. This condition is most commonly caused by inadequate production of testosterone and müllerian-inhibiting factor (MIF) by the fetal testes. The low testosterone and MIF levels will stunt the development of the male genitalia.

4–E. The most common cause of testicular feminization syndrome is the lack of androgen receptors in the urethral folds and genital swellings. Because these tissues lack androgen receptors, they are blind or unresponsive to androgens. Consequently, these tissues develop into female external genitalia even though the fetus has a 46,XY genotype.

5–A. Failure of the urethral folds to fuse completely results in the external urethral orifice opening onto the ventral surface of the penis, a condition known as hypospadias.

6–C. The gene product that is coded on the short arm of the Y chromosome is called the testes-determining factor (TDF).

7–B. Sterility is a common result of bilateral cryptorchidism. When both testes fail to descend into the scrotum, the increased temperature they are exposed to in the abdominal cavity will inhibit spermatogenesis.

8–A. This is a classic case of testicular feminization syndrome. A karyotype analysis would reveal that this normal-appearing 17-year-old girl actually has a 46,XY genotype. The mobile masses within the right and left labia majora are the testes and should be surgically removed because this tissue has a propensity toward malignant tumor formation. The most common cause of this syndrome is a lack of androgen receptors in the urethral folds and genital swellings.

9–A. A vestigial remnant of the paramesonephric duct called the appendix testis can sometimes be found in the male.

10–C. The efferent ductules that connect the rete testes with the epididymis are derived from the mesonephric tubules.

11–B. The epididymis is a mesonephric duct derivative.

12–B. The ductus deferens is a mesonephric duct derivative.

13–D. The glans penis is a phallus derivative.

14–F. The scrotum is derived from the genital swellings.

15–B. The seminal vesicle is a mesonephric duct derivative.

16–E. The penile raphe is a scar-like line made up of surface ectoderm found along the ventral surface of the penis. It is formed when the urethral folds fuse, thereby bringing together the surface ectoderm.

17–B. The ejaculatory duct is a mesonephric duct derivative.

16

Integumentary System

I. Skin

– is the largest organ of the body, with a surface area of approximately 2 m².
– functions as a barrier against infection, serves thermoregulation, and protects the body against dehydration.

A. Epidermis

– is derived from the ectoderm.

1. Early development

– The epidermis consists of a single layer of ectodermal cells that give rise to an overlying **periderm** layer.
– The epidermis soon becomes a three-layered structure consisting of the stratum basale (mitotically active), intermediate layer (progeny of stratum basale), and the periderm.
– Peridermal cells are eventually desquamated and form part of the **vernix caseosa**, a greasy substance of peridermal cells and sebum from the sebaceous glands that protects the embryo's skin.

2. Later development

– The definitive adult layers are formed, which depends upon the inductive influence of the dermis.

a. Stratum basale

b. Stratum spinosum

c. Stratum granulosum

d. Stratum corneum

3. Other cells of the epidermis

a. Melanoblasts

– are derived from **neural crest** and migrate into the stratum basale of the epidermis.
– differentiate into melanocytes by mid-pregnancy when pigment granules called **melanosomes** are observed.

193

b. Langerhans cells

– are derived from the bone marrow (mesoderm) and migrate into the epidermis.

– are involved in antigen presentation.

c. Merkel cells

– are of uncertain origin and migrate into the epidermis.

– are associated with free nerve endings and probably function as mechanoreceptors.

B. Dermis

– is derived from both the somatic mesoderm located just beneath the ectoderm and the mesoderm of the dermatomes in most of the body.

– is derived from neural crest cells in the head and neck region (see Chapter 12).

1. Early development

– is initially composed of loosely aggregated mesodermal cells frequently referred to as mesenchymal cells (or mesenchyme).

– The mesenchymal cells secrete a watery-type extracellular matrix rich in glycogen and hyaluronic acid.

2. Later development

– Mesenchymal cells differentiate into fibroblasts which secrete increasing amounts of collagen and elastic fibers into the extracellular matrix.

– Vascularization occurs.

– Sensory nerves grow into the dermis.

– Forms projections into the epidermis called dermal papillae, which contain tactile sensory receptors, such as Meissner's corpuscles.

C. Clinical considerations

1. Albinism

– is an autosomal recessive trait.

– results when melanocytes **fail to produce melanin** in the skin, hair, and eyes.

– is caused by a lack of the enzyme **tyrosinase**.

– predisposes to basal and squamous cell carcinoma, and malignant melanoma.

2. Hemangiomas

– are vascular malformations, benign tumors of endothelial cells.

– produce "birth marks" (e.g., **port-wine stain**, frequently associated with the Sturge-Weber syndrome).

3. Ichthyosis

– is an X-linked disorder of keratinization, characterized by dryness and scaling of the skin.

4. Psoriasis

– is a skin disease characterized by **excess cell proliferation** in the stratum basale and in the stratum spinosum, resulting in thickening of the epidermis and shorter regeneration time of the epidermis.

5. Ehlers-Danlos syndrome
  – is a genetic defect involving **peptidyl lysine hydroxylase**, which is necessary for the hydroxylation of lysine residues of collagen.
  – affects mainly **Type I** and **Type III collagen**.
  – is characterized by skin that is extremely stretchable, fragile, and vulnerable to injury.

II. Hair and Nails

– are derived from ectoderm.

A. Hair
  – Cells from the stratum basale grow into the underlying dermis and form the **hair follicle**.
  – The deepest part of the hair follicle soon becomes club-shaped to form the **hair bulb**.
  – The hair bulbs are invaginated by mesodermal **hair papillae**, which are rapidly filled with blood vessels and nerve endings.
  – Epithelial cells within the hair bulb differentiate into the **germinal matrix** where cells proliferate, grow towards the surface, keratinize, and form the **hair shaft**. These cells also form the **internal root sheath**.
  – Other epithelial cells of the hair follicle form the **external root sheath**.
  – Mesodermal cells of the dermis that surround the invaginating hair follicle form the **dermal root sheath**.
  – Smooth muscle fibers, the **arrector pili muscle**, develop from the mesoderm and attach to the hair follicle.
  – The first fine hairs, called **lanugo hairs**, are sloughed off at birth.

B. Nails
  – develop from the epidermis.
  – first develop on the tips of the digits, then migrate to the dorsal surface, taking their innervation with them; this is why the median nerve innervates the dorsal tips of the index finger, middle finger, and one-half of the ring finger.

C. Clinical considerations

1. Alopecia
  – is baldness resulting from an absence or faulty development of the hair follicles.

2. Hypertrichosis
  – is an overgrowth of hair.
  – is frequently associated with spina bifida occulta; seen as a patch of hair overlying the defect.

3. Pili torti
  – is a familial disorder characterized by twisted hairs.
  – is seen in Menkes' (kinky-hair) disease, an X-linked recessive neurologic disorder.

III. Mammary, Sweat, and Sebaceous Glands

– are all derived from the surface ectoderm.

A. Mammary glands

– develop from the **mammary ridge**, a downgrowth of the epidermis (ectoderm) into the underlying dermis (mesoderm).
– Canalization of these epithelial sprouts results in formation of **alveoli** and **lactiferous ducts**; the latter drain into an epithelial pit, the future **nipple**.

B. Sweat glands

– develop from downgrowths of the epidermis into the underlying dermis.
– include **eccrine** and **apocrine glands**.

C. Sebaceous glands

– develop from the epithelial wall of the hair follicle and elaborate **sebum** into the hair follicles.
– The **tarsal (meibomian) glands** of the eyelids do not communicate with hair follicles.

D. Clinical considerations

1. Gynecomastia

– is a condition in which there is excessive development of the male mammary glands.
– is frequently associated with Klinefelter's syndrome (47,XXY).

2. Polymastia

– is a condition in which supernumerary breasts occur along the mammary ridge.

3. Polythelia

– is a condition in which supernumerary nipples occur along the mammary ridge.

IV. Teeth (Figure 16-1)

– develop from ectoderm and an underlying layer of neural crest cells.

A. Dental lamina

– develops from the oral epithelium as a downgrowth into the underlying neural crest layer.
– gives rise to **tooth buds**, which develop into the **enamel organs**.

B. Enamel organs

– are derived from ectoderm.
– develop first for the 20 deciduous teeth, then for the 32 permanent teeth.
– give rise to **ameloblasts**, which produce **enamel**.

C. Dental papilla

– is formed by **neural crest** cells that underlie the enamel organ.
– gives rise to the **odontoblasts**, which produce **predentin** and **dentin**, and to the **dental pulp**.

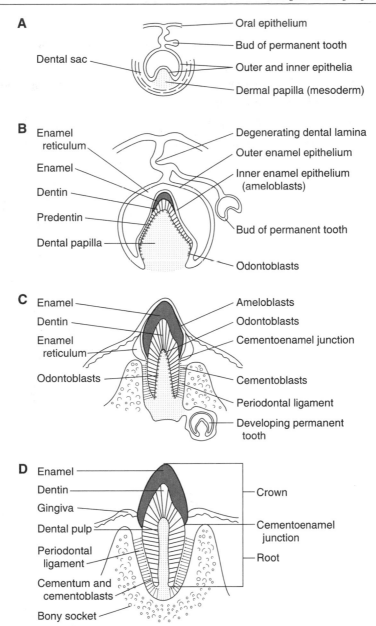

Figure 16–1. Schematic drawing showing successive stages in the development of a tooth. Ameloblasts give rise to enamel, and odontoblasts, of neural crest origin, give rise to dentin.

D. Dental sac

- is formed by a condensation of neural crest cells that surround the dental papilla.
- gives rise to **cementoblasts**, which form **cementum**, and to the **periodontal ligaments**.

E. Clinical considerations

1. Defective enamel formation (amelogenesis imperfecta)

– is an autosomal dominant trait.

2. Defective dentin formation (dentinogenesis imperfecta)

– is an autosomal dominant trait.

3. Discoloration of teeth

– is caused by the administration of **tetracyclines**, which stain and affect the enamel of both deciduous and permanent teeth.

Review Test

Directions: Each of the numbered items or incomplete statements in this section is followed by answers or by completions of the statement. Select the **one** lettered answer or completion that is **best** in each case.

1. Melanocytes are found in which epidermal layer?

(A) Stratum basale
(B) Stratum corneum
(C) Stratum granulosum
(D) Stratum lucidum
(E) Stratum spinosum

2. All of the following structures are derived from the epidermis EXCEPT

(A) hair follicles
(B) nails
(C) the mammary ridge
(D) melanocytes
(E) sebaceous glands

3. The dental lamina gives rise to all of the following structures EXCEPT

(A) the dental papilla
(B) the enamel organ
(C) tooth buds for deciduous teeth
(D) tooth buds for permanent teeth
(E) ameloblasts

4. All of the following statements concerning albinism are correct EXCEPT

(A) it results from a lack of the enzyme tyrosinase
(B) it is most commonly an X-linked recessive trait
(C) it results when melanocytes fail to produce melanin in the skin, hair, and eyes
(D) it predisposes to basal and squamous cell carcinoma
(E) it predisposes to malignant melanoma

5. The administration of which of the following agents may result in discoloration of both deciduous and permanent teeth?

(A) Cephalosporin
(B) Chloramphenicol
(C) Erythromycin
(D) Penicillin
(E) Tetracycline

Answers and Explanations

1–A. Melanocytes are found in the stratum basale, the deepest layer of the epidermis, at the dermoepidermal junction.

2–D. Melanocytes are derived from the neural crest. The mammary ridge is a downgrowth of epidermis into the dermis, which forms the mammary glands.

3–A. The dental papilla is formed by the underlying layer of neural crest cells. It gives rise to odontoblasts, which produce predentin and dentin; it also gives rise to dental pulp.

4–B. Albinism is most commonly an autosomal recessive trait; there is a rare X-linked form of albinism.

5–E. Tetracyclines are bound to calcium in newly formed teeth both in utero and in young children. They may cause fluorescence, discoloration, and enamel dysplasia.

17
Skeletal System

I. Skull (Figures 17-1 and 17-2)

– The skull can be divided into two parts: the neurocranium and viscerocranium.

A. Neurocranium

– consists of the flat bones of the skull (cranial vault) and the base of the skull.

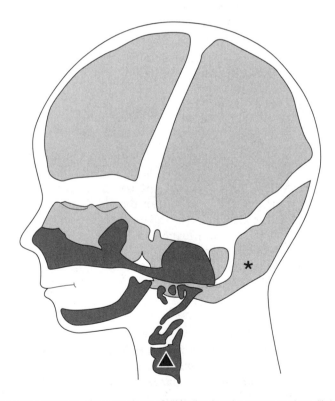

Figure 17–1. A schematic diagram of the newborn skull indicating the neurocranium *(lighter shaded area)* and the viscerocranium *(darker shaded area)*. The bones of the neurocranium and viscerocranium are derived almost entirely from neural crest cells, except for the basilar part of the occipital bone (*), which forms from mesoderm of the occipital sclerotomes, and the laryngeal cartilages (▲), which form from mesoderm within pharyngeal arches 4 and 6.

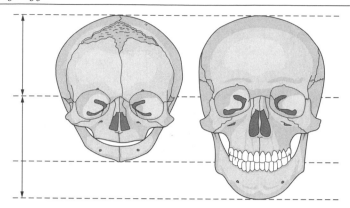

Figure 17–2. A schematic diagram depicting the postnatal growth of the skull. After birth, the skull continues ossification towards the sutures. However, the face is relatively underdeveloped and undergoes dramatic changes during childhood and adolescence with the eruption of teeth, formation of sinuses, and elongation of the maxilla and mandible. Note that the profound postnatal changes of the skull are due to the development of the viscerocranium. (Redrawn with permission from *Gray's Anatomy: The Anatomical Basis of Medicine and Surgery,* 38th ed. Edinburgh, Scotland, Churchill Livingstone, 1995, p. 372.)

  – develops from neural crest cells except for the basilar part of the occipital bone, which forms from mesoderm of the occipital sclerotomes.

B. Viscerocranium

  – consists of the bones of the face involving the pharyngeal arches, which have been discussed in Chapter 12.
  – develops from neural crest cells except for the laryngeal cartilages, which form from mesoderm within pharyngeal arches #4 and #6.

C. Sutures

  – During fetal life and infancy, the flat bones of the skull are separated by dense connective tissue (fibrous joints) called sutures.
  – There are five sutures: **frontal suture, sagittal suture, lambdoid suture, coronal suture**, and **squamosal suture.**
  – Sutures allow the flat bones of the skull to deform during childbirth (called **molding**) and to expand during childhood as the brain grows.
  – Molding may exert considerable tension at the "obstetrical hinge" (junction of the squamous and lateral parts of the occipital bone) such that the **great cerebral vein (of Galen)** is ruptured during childbirth.

D. Fontanelles

  – are large fibrous areas where several sutures meet.
  – There are six fontanelles: **anterior fontanelle, posterior fontanelle**, two **sphenoid fontanelles**, and two **mastoid fontanelles**.
  – The anterior fontanelle is the largest fontanelle and readily palpable in the infant. It pulsates because of the underlying cerebral arteries and can be used to obtain a blood sample from the underlying superior sagittal sinus. The anterior fontanelle and the mastoid fontanelles close at about **2 years of age** when the main growth of the brain ceases.
  – The posterior fontanelle and the sphenoid fontanelles close at about **6 months of age**.

E. Clinical considerations

1. Abnormalities in skull shape

– may result from failure of cranial sutures to form or from premature closure of sutures (craniosynostoses).

a. Microcephaly

– results from failure of the brain to grow; usually associated with mental retardation.

b. Oxycephaly (turricephaly or acrocephaly)

– is a tower-like skull caused by premature closure of the lambdoid and coronal sutures.
– **Crouzon's syndrome** is a dominant genetic condition that presents quite similarly to oxycephaly but is accompanied by malformations of the face, teeth, and ears.

c. Plagiocephaly

– is an asymmetric skull caused by premature closure of the lambdoid and coronal sutures on one side of the skull.

d. Scaphocephaly

– is a long, narrow skull (in the anterior/posterior plane) caused by premature closure of the sagittal suture.

2. Temporal bone formation

a. Mastoid process

– is absent at birth and forms by 2 years of age.
– This leaves the facial nerve (CN VII) relatively unprotected as it emerges from the stylomastoid foramen. In a difficult delivery, forceps may damage CN VII.

b. Petrosquamous fissure

– The petrous and squamous portions of the temporal bone are separated by the petrosquamous fissure, which opens directly into the mastoid antrum of the middle ear.
– This fissure may remain open until 20 years of age and provides a route for the spread of infection from the middle ear to the meninges.

3. Spheno-occipital joint

– is a site of growth up to about 20 years of age.

II. Vertebral Column

A. Vertebrae in general (Figure 17-3)

– Mesodermal cells from the sclerotome migrate and condense around the notochord to form the **centrum**, around the neural tube to form the **vertebral arches**, and in the body wall to form the **costal processes**.

1. Centrum: forms the vertebral body

2. Vertebral arches: form the pedicles, laminae, spinous process, articular processes, and the transverse processes

3. Costal processes: form the ribs

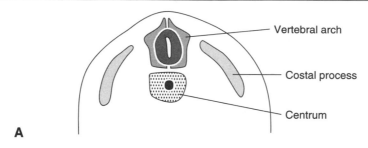

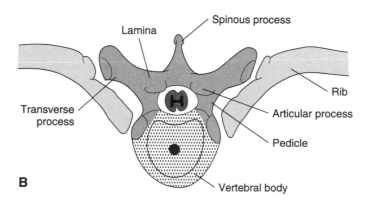

Figure 17–3. A schematic diagram indicating the development of a typical thoracic vertebra. *(A)* At about 5–7 weeks: Mesodermal cells from the sclerotome demonstrate three distinct condensations; centrum, vertebral arches, and costal processes. During 3–5 years of age, the vertebral arches fuse with each other and to the centrum. Ossification ends at about 25 years of age. *(B)* Adult: Each condensation develops into distinct components of the adult vertebrae as indicated by the *shading.*

B. Axis (C1) and Atlas (C2)

– are highly modified vertebrae.

1. The atlas has no vertebral body.

2. The axis has an **odontoid process (dens)** that represents the vertebral body of the atlas.

C. Sacrum

– is a large triangular fusion of five sacral vertebrae forming the posterior/superior wall of the pelvic cavity.

D. Coccyx

– is a small triangular fusion of four rudimentary vertebrae.

E. Intersegmental position of vertebrae (Figure 17-4)

– As mesodermal cells from the sclerotome migrate towards the notochord and neural tube, they split into a cranial portion and a caudal portion.

– The caudal portion of each sclerotome fuses with the cranial portion of the succeeding sclerotome, which results in the intersegmental position of the vertebra.

– The splitting of the sclerotome is important because it allows the developing spinal nerve a route of access to the myotome that it must innervate.

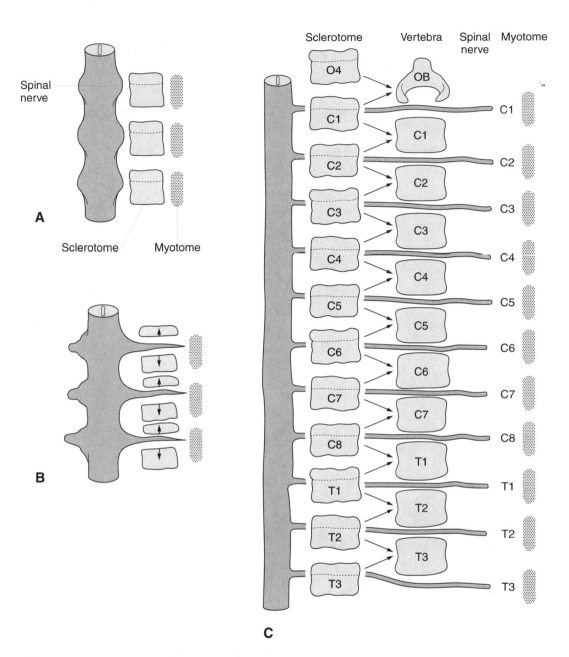

Figure 17-4. (*A* and *B*) Schematic diagram depicting the splitting of the sclerotome into caudal and cranial portions as the spinal nerves grow out to innervate the myotome. The dotted line in A indicates where the sclerotome splits, thus allowing the growing spinal nerve to reach the myotome. *(C)* Schematic diagram depicting the splitting of sclerotomes from the fourth occipital sclerome (O4) to the T3 sclerotome. Note that the caudal portion of O4 sclerotome fuses with the cranial portion of C1 sclerotome to form the base of the occipital bone. Also note that C1 spinal nerve exits between the base of the occipital bone and C1 vertebra. This diagram explains why there are eight cervical spinal nerves but only seven cervical vertebrae. *OB* = occipital bone. (Redrawn with permission from Larsen WJ: *Human Embryology,* 2nd ed. New York, Churchill Livingston, 1997, p 77.)

– In the cervical region, the caudal portion of the fourth occipital sclerotome (O4) fuses with the cranial portion of the first cervical (C1) sclerotome to form the base of the occipital bone, which allows the C1 spinal nerve to exit between the base of the occipital bone and C1 vertebra.

F. Curves

1. **Primary curves** are thoracic and sacral curvatures that form during the fetal period.

2. **Secondary curves** are cervical and lumbar curvatures that form after birth as a result of lifting the head and walking, respectively.

G. Joints of the vertebral column

1. **Synovial joints**

   a. **Atlanto-occipital joint**: between C1 (atlas) and the occipital condyles.

   b. **Atlanto-axial joint**: between C1 (atlas) and C2 (axis).

   c. **Facets (zygapophyseal) joints**: between the inferior and superior articular facets.

2. **Secondary cartilaginous joints (symphyses)**

   – are the joints between the vertebral bodies in which the intervertebral disks play a role.
   – An intervertebral disk consists of:

   a. **Nucleus pulposus**

      – is a remnant of the embryonic **notochord**.
      – By 20 years of age, all notochordal cells have degenerated such that all notochordal vestiges in the adult are limited to just a noncellular matrix.

   b. **Annulus fibrosus**

      – is an outer rim of fibrocartilage derived from mesoderm found between the vertebral bodies.

H. Clinical considerations (Figure 17-5)

1. **Congenital brevicollis (Klippel-Feil syndrome)**

   – results from fusion and shortening of the cervical vertebrae.
   – is associated with shortness of neck, low hairline, and limited motion of head and neck.

2. **Intervertebral disk herniation**

   – is prolapse of the **nucleus pulposus** through the **defective annulus fibrosus** into the vertebral canal.
   – The nucleus pulposus impinges on spinal roots and results in root pain, **radiculopathy**.

3. **Spina bifida occulta**

   – results from failure of the vertebral arches to form or fuse.

4. **Spondylolisthesis**

   – occurs when the pedicles of the vertebral arches fail to fuse with the vertebral body.

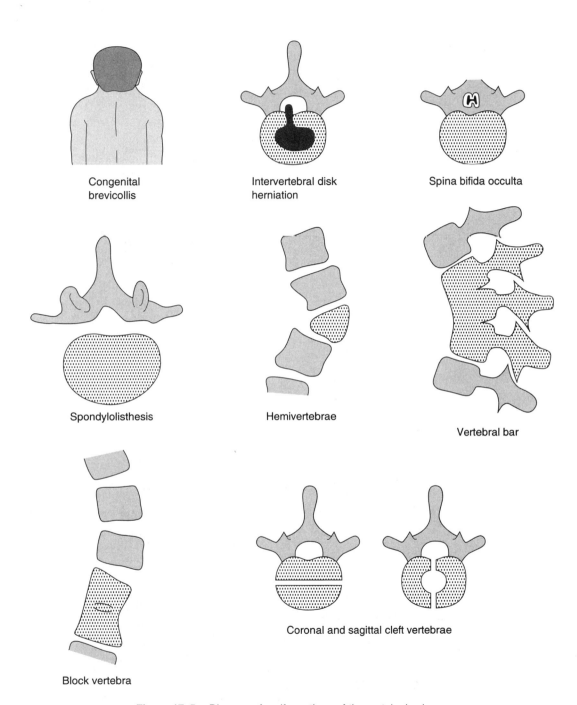

Congenital brevicollis

Intervertebral disk herniation

Spina bifida occulta

Spondylolisthesis

Hemivertebrae

Vertebral bar

Block vertebra

Coronal and sagittal cleft vertebrae

Figure 17–5. Diagram of malformations of the vertebral column.

– allows the vertebral body to move anterior with respect to the vertebra below it, causing lordosis.
– usually occurs in the lumbar region.

5. Hemivertebrae

– occurs when wedges of vertebrae appear that are usually situated laterally between two other vertebrae.

6. Vertebral bar

– occurs when there is a localized failure of segmentation on one side of the column, usually in a posterolateral site.

7. Block vertebra

– occurs when there is a lack of separation between two or more vertebrae, usually occurring in the lumbar region.

8. Cleft vertebra

– occurs when a cleft develops in the vertebra, usually in a coronal or sagittal plane in the lumbar region.

9. Idiopathic scoliosis

– is a lateral deviation of the vertebral column.
– involves both deviation and rotation of vertebral bodies.

III. Ribs

A. Development in general

– Ribs develop from costal processes, which form at all vertebral levels.
– However, only in the thoracic region do the costal processes grow into ribs.

B. Clinical considerations

1. Accessory lumbar ribs are the most common.

2. Accessory cervical ribs

– are attached to the C7 vertebra and may either end freely or be attached to the thoracic cage.
– may put pressure on the lower trunk of the brachial plexus and subclavian artery, causing **superior thoracic outlet syndrome**.

IV. Sternum

A. Development in general

– The sternum develops from two **sternal bars** that form in the ventral body wall independent of the ribs and clavicle.
– The sternal bars fuse with each other in a cranial–caudal direction to form the **manubrium, body**, and **xiphoid process** by week 8.

B. Clinical considerations

1. Sternal cleft

– occurs when the sternal bars do not fuse completely.
– is fairly common and if small is generally of no clinical significance.

2. Pectus excavatum (funnel chest)

- is the most common chest anomaly consisting of a depression of the chest wall that may extend from the manubrium to the xiphoid process.
- In addition to the cosmetic appearance, these individuals demonstrate cardiopulmonary restriction, drooped shoulders, protuberant abdomen, and scoliosis such that early surgical intervention is generally recommended.

3. Poland syndrome

- is a relatively uncommon chest anomaly characterized by the partial or complete absence of the **pectoralis major muscle**.
- In addition, these individuals may demonstrate partial agenesis of the ribs and ternum, mammary gland aplasia, or absence of the latissimus dorsi and serratus anterior muscles.

V. Bones of the Limbs and Limb Girdles

A. Development in general

- The bones of the limb and limb girdles develop from condensations of lateral plate mesoderm in the limb bud
- The limb buds are visible in week 4 of development; the upper limb appears first.
- The limbs are well differentiated at week 8.
- The limb tip contains the **apical ectodermal ridge**, which exerts an inductive influence on limb growth and development.

B. Clinical considerations

1. **Amelia** (an absence of one or two extremities) may have resulted from the use of the teratogen **thalidomide**.
2. **Polydactyly** is an autosomal dominant disorder characterized by the presence of **extra digits** on the hands or feet.
3. **Syndactyly** (webbed fingers or toes) is the most common limb anomaly; results from failure of the hand or foot webs to degenerate between the digits.
4. **Holt-Oram syndrome (Heart-Hand syndrome)** is an autosomal dominant condition associated with chromosome 12 that causes anomalies of the upper limb and heart.

VI. Osteogenesis: occurs by replacement of preexisting connective tissue (mesoderm). During development, two types of ossification occur.

A. Intramembranous ossification

- occurs in the embryo when mesoderm condenses into sheets of highly vascular **connective tissue**, which then directly forms a primary ossification center.
- Bones that form via intramembranous ossification are: frontal bone, parietal bones, intraparietal part of occipital bone, maxilla, zygomatic bone, squamous part of temporal bone, palatine, vomer, and mandible.

B. Endochondral ossification

- occurs in the embryo when mesoderm first forms a **hyaline cartilage** model, which then develops a primary ossification center at the diaphysis.

– Bones that form via endochondral ossification are: ethmoid bone, sphenoid bone, petrous and mastoid parts of the temporal bone, basilar part of the occipital bone, incus, malleus, stapes, styloid process, hyoid bone, bones of the limbs, limb girdles, vertebrae, sternum, and ribs.

VII. General Skeletal Abnormalities

A. Achondroplasia

– is an autosomal dominant disorder (**dwarfism**) characterized by large head, short stature, short limbs and fingers, and normal trunk.
– is the most prevalent form of dwarfism although the cause is not known.
– Pathologic changes are observed at the epiphyseal growth plate where the zones of proliferation and hypertrophy are narrow and disorganized; horizontal struts of bone eventually grow into the growth plate and "seal" the bone, thereby preventing bone growth.
– Mental function is not affected.
– Chances of achondroplasia increase with increasing paternal age.

B. Acromegaly

– results from **hyperpituitarism**.
– is characterized by a large jaw, hands, and feet, and sometimes by **gigantism**.

C. Osteogenesis imperfecta

– is caused by a deficiency in **Type I collagen**.
– is characterized by extreme bone fragility, with spontaneous fractures occurring when the fetus is still in the womb, and blue sclera of the eye
– is fatal in utero or during the early neonatal period.

D. Marfan syndrome

– is a genetic defect involving the protein **fibrillin**, which is an essential component of elastic fibers.
– These individuals are unusually tall and have exceptionally long limbs and ectopia lentis (dislocation of the lens).

E. Cretinism

– occurs when there is a deficiency in fetal **thyroid hormone (T_3 and T_4)** and/or **thyroid agenesis**.
– results in growth retardation, skeletal abnormalities, mental retardation, and neurologic disorders.
– is rare except in areas where there is a lack of iodine in the water and soil.

Review Test

Directions: Each of the numbered items or incomplete statements in this section is followed by answers or by completions of the statement. Select the **one** lettered answer or completion that is **best** in each case.

1. Accessory ribs are most commonly found attached to the

(A) cervical vertebrae
(B) thoracic vertebrae
(C) lumbar vertebrae
(D) manubrium
(E) sternebrae

2. The anterior fontanelle is usually closed by

(A) birth
(B) age 6 months
(C) age 18 months
(D) age 2 years
(E) age 5 years

3. The condition where the pedicles of the vertebral arches fail to fuse with the vertebral body is called

(A) block vertebrae
(B) cleft vertebrae
(C) hemivertebrae
(D) spondylolisthesis
(E) spina bifida occulta

4. During ultrasound examination, numerous fractures of the long bones of the fetus are observed. This condition is called

(A) achondroplasia
(B) osteogenesis imperfecta
(C) Marfan syndrome
(D) cretinism
(E) acromegaly

Directions: Each group of items in this section consists of lettered options followed by a set of numbered items. For each item, select the **one** lettered option that is most closely associated with it. Each lettered option may be selected once, more than once, or not at all.

Questions 5–9

Match each description below with the appropriate skeletal malformation.

(A) Achondroplasia
(B) Acromegaly
(C) Oxycephaly
(D) Plagiocephaly
(E) Scaphocephaly

5. Results from premature closure of the sagittal suture

6. Results from premature closure of the coronal suture

7. Results from premature closure of sutures on one side of the skull

8. A result of hyperpituitarism

9. Retardation of epiphyseal growth

Answers and Explanations

1–C. Accessory ribs are most commonly attached to lumbar vertebrae. When present (incidence 0.5%–1%), a cervical rib is usually attached to the seventh cervical vertebra. Cervical ribs may compress the brachial plexus and subclavian vessels and cause superior thoracic outlet syndrome.

2–D. The anterior fontanelle is usually closed by 2 years of age; the posterior and sphenoid fontanelles are usually closed by 6 months of age.

3–D. When the pedicles fail to fuse with the vertebral body, a condition called spondylolisthesis results. This allows the vertebral body to move anterior with respect to the vertebra below it, causing lordosis.

4–B. Osteogenesis imperfecta is a deficiency of Type I collagen and results in spontaneous fractures of fetal bones and blue sclera of the eye.

5–E. Scaphocephaly, or tectocephaly, is a long narrow skull resulting from premature closure of the sagittal suture; it is a form of craniosynostosis.

6–C. Oxycephaly, or acrocephaly, is a steeple or tower skull resulting from lack of the coronal and lambdoid sutures; it is a form of craniosynostosis.

7–D. Plagiocephaly is an asymmetric craniosynostosis caused by premature closure of sutures on one side of the head (the lambdoid and coronal sutures). It is an oblique deformity of the skull.

8–B. Acromegaly results from hyperpituitarism with excessive secretion of somatotropin. It is characterized by progressive enlargement of peripheral parts of the body, especially the head, face, hands, and feet.

9–A. Achondroplasia is caused by retardation of epiphyseal growth. This results in dwarfism with short extremities.

18

Muscular System

I. Skeletal Muscle

A. Paraxial mesoderm

- is a thick plate of mesoderm on each side of the midline.
- becomes organized into segments known as **somitomeres**, which form in a craniocaudal sequence.
- Somitomeres 1–7 do not form somites but contribute mesoderm to the head and neck region **(pharyngeal arches)**.
- The remaining somitomeres further condense in a craniocaudal sequence to form **42–44 pairs of somites** of the trunk region.
- The somites closest to the caudal end eventually disappear to give a final count of approximately 35 pairs of somites.
- Somites further differentiate into the **sclerotome** (cartilage and bone component), **myotome** (muscle component), and **dermatome** (dermis of skin component).

B. Head and neck musculature (see Chapter 12)

- is derived from somitomeres 1–7 of the head and neck region, which participate in the formation of the pharyngeal arches.

1. Extraocular muscles

- are derived from somitomeres 1, 2, 3, and 5.
- Somitomeres 1, 2, and 3 are called **preotic myotomes (somites)**.
- are innervated by CN III, CN IV, and CN VI.

2. Tongue muscles

- are derived from the myotomes in the occipital region.
- are innervated by CN XII.

C. Trunk musculature (Figure 18-1)

- is derived from myotomes in the trunk region that partition into dorsal **epimeres** and ventral **hypomeres**.

1. Epimeres

- develop into the intrinsic back muscles (e.g., erector spinae).
- are innervated by the **dorsal rami** of spinal nerves.

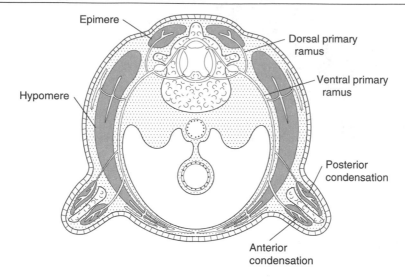

Figure 18-1. Schematic drawing of a transverse section through the thorax and limb bud, showing the muscles of the epimere, hypomere, and the limb bud. The limb bud musculature develops from mesoderm of various myotomes. The epimeric muscles are innervated by dorsal primary rami, and the hypomeric and limb muscles are innervated by ventral primary rami of spinal nerves.

    2. Hypomeres
        – develop into the prevertebral, intercostal, and abdominal muscles.
        – are innervated by the **ventral rami** of spinal nerves.

D. Limb musculature (see Figure 18-1)
    – is derived from myotomes (somites) in the upper limb bud region and lower limb bud region.
    – This mesoderm migrates into the limb bud and forms a **posterior condensation** and an **anterior condensation**.

    1. Posterior condensation
        – develops into the **extensor** and **supinator** musculature of the upper limb
        – develops into the **extensor** and **abductor** musculature of the lower limb.

    2. Anterior condensation
        – develops into the **flexor** and **pronator** musculature of the upper limb
        – develops into the **flexor** and **adductor** musculature of the lower limb.

II. Smooth Muscle

    – of the gastrointestinal (GI) tract and the tunica media of blood vessels is derived from mesoderm.

III. Cardiac Muscle

    – is derived from mesoderm, which surrounds the primitive heart tube and becomes the myocardium.

Review Test

Directions: The group of items in this section consists of lettered options followed by a set of numbered items. For each item, select the **one** lettered option that is most closely associated with it. Each lettered option may be selected once, more than once, or not at all.

Questions 1–5

Match each muscle group with the appropriate structure of origin.

(A) Cervical somites
(B) Epimere
(C) Hypomere
(D) Occipital somites
(E) Preotic somites

1. Abdominal muscles

2. Extrinsic eye muscles

3. Erector spinae muscle

4. Tongue muscles

5. Septum transversum

Directions: Each of the numbered items or incomplete statements in this section is followed by answers or by completions of the statement. Select the **one** lettered answer or completion that is **best** in each case.

6. The biceps brachii muscle develops from which of the following?

(A) Hypomere
(B) Epimere
(C) Anterior condensation
(D) Posterior condensation
(E) Preotic somites

7. The biceps femoris muscle develops from which of the following?

(A) Hypomere
(B) Epimere
(C) Anterior condensation
(D) Posterior condensation
(E) Preotic somites

Answers and Explanations

1–C. The hypomere (ventral part of the myotome) gives rise to the flexor muscles of the neck and vertebral column, the intercostal muscles, the abdominal muscles, and the muscles of the pelvic diaphragm.

2–E. The extrinsic eye muscles arise from the preotic somites (myotomes) found near the prochordal plate. Recent research indicates that the extrinsic eye muscles are derived from somitomeres 1, 2, 3, and 5.

3–B. The epimere (dorsal part of the myotome) gives rise to the extensor muscles of the vertebral column, such as the erector spinae.

4–D. The tongue muscles (intrinsic and extrinsic) arise from the occipital somites (myotomes).

5–A. The septum transversum forms the muscle and central tendon of the diaphragm; it develops from the cervical somites (myotomes). The diaphragm is innervated by the phrenic nerve, which arises from C3 to C5. Its costal rim receives sensory fibers from lower intercostal (thoracic) nerves.

6–C. Since the biceps brachii muscle is a flexor of the antebrachium (forearm), it develops from the anterior condensation of myotomic mesoderm.

7–C. Since the biceps femoris muscle is a flexor of the leg, it develops from the anterior condensation of myotomic mesoderm.

19
Upper Limb Development

I. Upper Limb Development in General

A. Begins with the activation of a group of mesodermal cells of the **lateral plate mesoderm**
   - Lateral plate mesoderm migrates into the limb bud and condenses along the central axis to eventually form the **vasculature** and **skeletal** components of the upper limb.

B. Mesoderm from the somites
   - also migrates into the limb bud and condenses to eventually form the **musculature** components of the upper limb.

C. Future limb mesodermal cells
   - express the homeobox gene **Hox 3.3** before there is any hint of limb bud formation.

D. Limb mesoderm
   - signals ectoderm at the tip of the limb bud to thicken and form the **apical ectodermal ridge (AER)**.

E. Apical ectodermal ridge (AER)
   - interacts with underlying mesoderm to promote outgrowth of the limb bud by promoting mitosis and preventing terminal differentiation of mesodermal cells at the tip of the limb bud.

F. Zone of polarizing activity (ZPA)
   - consists of mesodermal cells located at the base of the limb bud.
   - directs the organization of the limb bud and patterning of the digits, both of which involve **retinoic acid (vitamin A)** and homeobox gene **Hox-4**.

G. Digit formation
   - occurs as a result of selected **apoptosis** within the AER such that five separate regions of AER remain at the tips of the future digits.

II. Vasculature (Figure 19-1)

A. Aortic arch #4

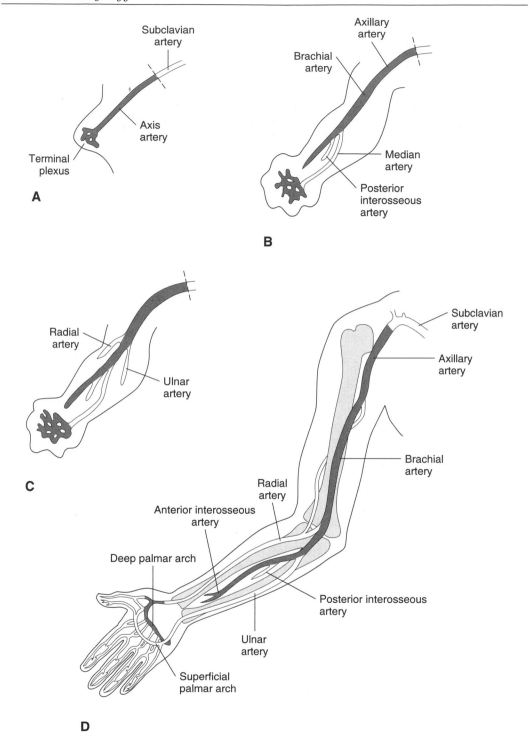

Figure 19-1. Diagram depicting the development of arteries of the upper limb. *(A, B, C)* Early limb bud. The earliest arterial supply of the upper limb bud is the axis artery *(dark shading)* and terminal plexus *(dark shading)*. The first branches of the axis artery are the posterior interosseous artery and the median artery. The last branches of the axis artery are the radial artery and ulnar artery. *(D)* Adult upper limb. The axis artery persists as the axillary artery, brachial artery, and anterior interosseous artery *(dark shading)*. Bones *(light shading)*.

– forms the proximal part of the right subclavian artery.

B. 7th intersegmental artery

– forms the distal part of the right subclavian artery.
– forms the entire left subclavian artery.

C. Subclavian artery (right and left)

– continues into the limb bud as the **axis artery**, which ends in a **terminal plexus** near the tip of the limb bud.

D. Terminal plexus

– participates in the formation of the **deep palmar arch** and **superficial palmar arch**.

E. Axis artery

1. First forms the **posterior interosseous artery** and the **median artery** (which is eventually reduced to a small unnamed vessel)

2. Last forms the **radial artery** and **ulnar artery**
   – The radial artery links with the terminal plexus to form the deep palmar arch.
   – The ulnar artery links with the terminal plexus to form the superficial palmar arch.

3. Ultimately persists in the adult as the **axillary artery, brachial artery, anterior interosseous artery,** and **deep palmar arch**.

III. Skeletal (Figure 19-2)

A. Lateral plate mesoderm

– forms the scapula, clavicle, humerus, radius, ulna, carpals, metacarpals, and phalanges.

B. All bones of the upper limb undergo endochondral ossification

C. Clavicle undergoes both membranous and endochondral ossification

D. Timing of bone formation

1. Week 5: Lateral plate mesoderm within the limb bud condenses

2. Week 6: Condensed mesoderm chondrifies to form a hyaline cartilage model of the upper limb bones

3. Week 7: Primary ossification centers seen in the clavicle, humerus, radius, and ulnar bones
   – The clavicle is the first bone in the entire body to ossify.

4. Week 9 to birth: Primary ossification centers seen in the scapula, metacarpals, and phalanges

5. Childhood: Secondary ossification centers form in the epiphyseal ends
   – All carpal bones begin ossification.

Week 5

Week 6

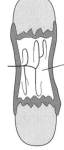

Primary
ossification
center

Weeks 7–9

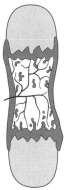

At birth

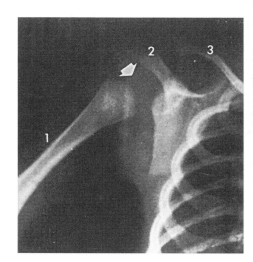

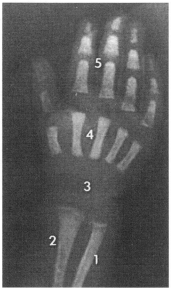

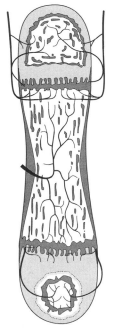

Childhood

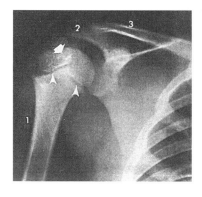

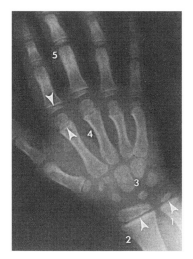

IV. Musculature (Figure 19-3 and 19-4)

A. Upper limb bud site

1. Lies opposite somites C4, C5, C6, C7, C8, T1, and T2

2. During week 5, mesoderm from these somites (myotomes) migrates into the limb bud and forms a **posterior condensation** and an **anterior condensation**

   a. The mesoderm of these condensations differentiates into myoblasts; then the condensations split into anatomically recognizable muscles of the upper limb, although little is known about this process

   b. **Posterior condensation** gives rise to these specific muscles: deltoid, supraspinatus, infraspinatus, teres minor, teres major, subscapularis, triceps brachii, anconeus, brachioradialis, extensor carpi radialis longus, extensor carpi radialis brevis, extensor digitorum, extensor digiti minimi, extensor carpi ulnaris, supinator, abductor pollicis longus, extensor pollicis brevis, extensor pollicis longus, and extensor indicis; in general, the **extensor** and **supinator** musculature.

   c. **Anterior condensation** gives rise to these specific muscles: biceps brachii, brachialis, coracobrachialis, pronator teres, flexor carpi radialis, palmaris longus, flexor carpi ulnaris, flexor digitorum superficialis, flexor digitorum profundus, flexor pollicis brevis, flexor pollicis longus, pronator quadratus, abductor pollicis brevis, opponens pollicis, adductor pollicis, abductor digiti minimi, flexor digiti minimi brevis, opponens digiti minimi, lumbricals, dorsal and palmar interossei; in general, the **flexor** and **pronator** musculature.

Figure 19-2. Bone formation in upper limb. **Week 5.** Lateral plate mesoderm condenses (*hatched*). **Week 6.** Hyaline cartilage (*light shading*) model of future bones forms. **Weeks 7 to 9.** Primary ossification centers within the diaphysis appear such that bone (*dark shading*) forms (osteogenesis). **At birth:** The diaphysis consists of bone (*dark shading*), whereas the epiphysis remains hyaline cartilage (*light shading*). This is important to note when interpreting radiographs of newborns. The radiograph of a newborn at the shoulder region (*1* = humerus; *2* = acromion; *3* = clavicle) shows the portion of the hyaline cartilage model that has been replaced by radiodense bone (white). Note that the epiphyseal end of the humerus (white arrow) is still hyaline cartilage at birth and therefore will appear radiolucent (dark). The radiograph of a newborn arm and hand shows the portion of the hyaline cartilage model that has been replaced by radiodense bone (white) in the ulnar (*1*), radius (*2*), metacarpals (*4*), and phalanges (*5*). Note that the epiphyseal ends of these bones (*1, 2, 4, 5*) and all of the carpal bones (*3*) are still hyaline cartilage and therefore radiolucent (dark). The carpel bones of the wrist begin to ossify much later in childhood. **Childhood:** During childhood, secondary ossification centers form in the epiphyseal ends of the bones. During childhood and adolescence, the growth in length of long bones occurs at the epiphyseal growth plate. Note the radiograph of a 6-year-old child at the shoulder region (*1* = humerus; *2* = acromion; *3* = clavicle). Since secondary ossification centers are present within the epiphyseal ends of the humerus, the head of the humerus is now radiodense (*white arrow*), and the epiphyseal growth plate (*arrowheads*), where hyaline cartilage is present, remains radiolucent (dark). This is not to be confused with bone fracture. The radiograph of a 6-year-old child at the wrist and hand demonstrates the radiodense bone (white) within the diaphyseal and epiphyseal growth plates (*arrowheads*) which are hyaline cartilage. The diaphyseal and epiphyseal portions of the metacarpals (*4*) and phalanges (*5*) as well as their epiphyseal growth plates (arrowheads) can also be observed. Note that the carpal bones (*3*) have begun to ossify. (Radiographs reprinted from Keats TE, Smith TH: *An Atlas of Normal Developmental Roentgen Anatomy*, 2nd ed. Chicago, Year Book Medical Publishers, 1977, pp 33, 292, and 295.)

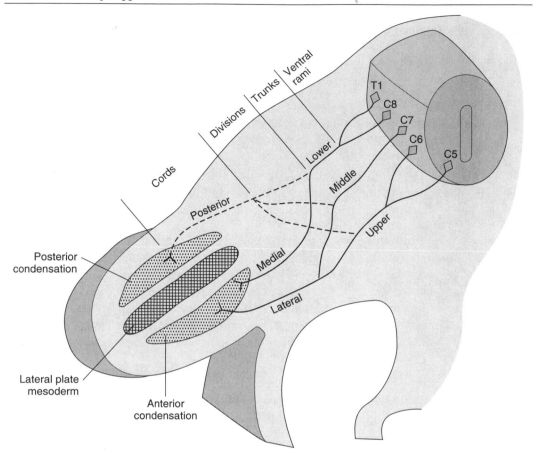

Figure 19-3. Diagram of the muscle and nerve development of the upper limb. Lateral plate mesoderm *(hatched area)* forms down the central axis of the limb bud and is responsible for the formation of the blood vessels and bones of the upper limb. Mesoderm from the somites (myotomes) migrates into the limb bud and forms a posterior and anterior condensation *(dotted areas)*. Ventral primary rami from C5 to T1 leave the neural tube and undergo extensive rearrangement into upper, middle ,and lower trunks. Each trunk divides into posterior *(dotted lines)* and anterior *(solid lines)* divisions. The posterior divisions selectively grow into the posterior condensation and form the posterior cord. The anterior divisions selectively grow into the anterior condensation and form the medial and lateral cords.

V. Nerves (Brachial Plexus) (see Figure 19-3)

A. Early nerve fibers

– are guided into the limb bud by local cell biological messages at its base; the muscles themselves do not provide any specific target messages to the ingrowing nerve fibers.

B. Ventral primary rami from C5, C6, C7, C8, and T1

1. Arrive at the base of the limb bud and join in a specific pattern to form the **upper trunk, middle trunk,** and **lower trunk**

2. Each trunk will divide into **posterior divisions** and **anterior divisions**

   a. Posterior divisions grow into the posterior condensation of mesoderm and join to form the **posterior cord**

– The **posterior cord,** with further development of the limb musculature, will branch into the **axillary nerve (C5, C6)** and **radial nerve (C5, C6, C7, C8, T1),** thereby innervating all the muscles that form from the posterior condensation.

   b. Anterior divisions grow into the anterior condensation of mesoderm and join to form the **medial cord** and **lateral cord**

     – The **medial cord** and **lateral cord,** with further development of the limb musculature, will branch into the **musculocutaneous nerve (C5, C6, C7), ulnar nerve (C8, T1), and median nerve (C5, C6, C7, C8, T1),** thereby innervating all the muscles that form from the anterior condensation.

VI. Rotation (Figure 19-4)

A. Upper limb buds

– appear in week 4 as small bulges oriented in a **coronal plane.**

– undergo a horizontal flexion in week 6 so that they are now oriented in a **parasagittal plane.**

B. Upper limbs

– **rotate laterally 90°** during weeks 6 to 8 such that the elbow points posteriorly, the extensor compartment lies posterior, and the flexor compartment lies anterior.

– This rotation causes the originally straight segmental pattern of innervation (dermatomes) to be somewhat modified in the adult.

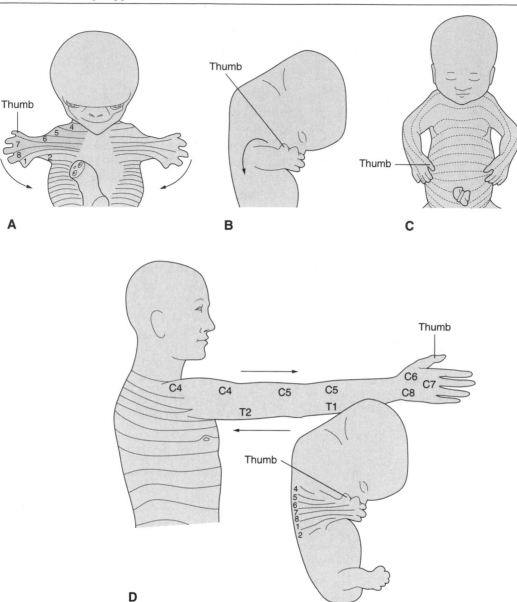

Figure 19-4. Rotation of the upper limb. *(A)* Ventral view of a week 4 embryo. Upper limb buds are oriented in a coronal plane. Note the segmental pattern of innervation from C4 to T2. In week 6, the upper limb buds undergo a horizontal flexion *(curved arrows)* such that the upper limb buds become oriented in a parasagittal plane (as shown in *B*). *(B)* Side view of a week 6 embryo. Note the upper limb bud oriented in the parasagittal plane. During weeks 6 to 8, the upper limb buds rotate 90° laterally *(curved arrow)*. *(C)* Ventral view of a week 8 embryo. Note the position of the upper limb with elbows pointing posterior. *(D)* Dermatome pattern in the adult upper limb and limb bud. The 90° lateral rotation of the upper limb bud causes the originally straight segmental pattern of innervation in the embryo to be somewhat modified ("twisted in a spiral") such that the dermatome pattern in the adult is altered. However, an orderly dermatome pattern can still be recognized in the adult if the upper limb is positioned in the parasagittal plane with the thumb pointing superiorly (as shown). The dermatomes from C4 can be counted distally down the superior border of the upper limb *(arrow)* to C7 at the middle finger and then back proximally up the inferior border of the upper limb *(arrow)* to T2. Note the position of the thumb in *A, B, C,* and *D*. (*A:* Redrawn with permission from Sadler TW: *Langman's Medical Embryology,* 7th ed. Baltimore, Williams & Wilkins, 1996, p 170. *C:* Redrawn with permission from Larson WJ: *Human Embryology,* 2nd ed. New York, Churchill Livingstone, 1997, p 323.)

Review Test

Directions: Each of the numbered items or incomplete statements in this section is followed by answers or by completions of the statement. Select the **one** lettered answer or completion that is **best** in each case.

1. Which of the following arteries is one of the first branches to form from the axis artery?

(A) radial artery
(B) ulnar artery
(C) axillary artery
(D) median artery
(E) brachial artery

2. The humerus develops from which of the following?

(A) somite mesoderm
(B) lateral plate mesoderm
(C) intermediate mesoderm
(D) extraembryonic mesoderm
(E) sclerotome mesoderm

3. The long head of the triceps muscle develops from which of the following?

(A) posterior condensation
(B) anterior condensation
(C) lateral plate mesoderm
(D) extraembryonic mesoderm
(E) sclerotome mesoderm

4. Which of the following muscles will the lateral cord of the brachial plexus innervate?

(A) triceps
(B) supinator
(C) extensor carpi ulnaris
(D) extensor digitorum
(E) biceps brachii

5. During weeks 6 to 8, the upper limb will rotate

(A) medially 90°
(B) laterally 90°
(C) medially 180°
(D) laterally 180°
(E) No rotation occurs

Answers and Explanations

1–D. The median artery is one of the first branches to form from the axis artery. In the adult, the median artery does not persist and is probably reduced to a small unnamed vessel. This is why the median nerve does not have an accompanying artery in the adult like the ulnar nerve (ulnar artery) and radial nerve (radial artery).

2–B. All bones of the upper limb form from lateral plate mesoderm that condenses along the central axis of the upper limb bud.

3–A. Somite mesoderm migrates into the limb bud and forms two condensations. The posterior condensation of the upper limb gives rise to the extensors of the upper limb, which attain a posterior location in the adult because of the lateral rotation of 90°.

4–E. One of the nerves that forms from the lateral cord of the brachial plexus is the musculocutaneous nerve. The musculocutaneous nerve will innervate muscles derived from the anterior condensation (flexors). Biceps brachii muscle is a flexor at the elbow joint. Note that the biceps brachii muscle and the musculocutaneous nerve are related embryologically to the anterior condensation and anterior divisions (which form the lateral cord) and in the adult are located anterior. This occurs because of the lateral rotation of 90°.

5–B. The upper limb rotates laterally 90° so that the elbows point posteriorly.

20
Lower Limb Development

I. Lower Limb Development in General

A. Begins with the activation of a group of mesodermal cells of the **lateral plate mesoderm**
 – Lateral plate mesoderm migrates into the limb bud and condenses along the central axis to eventually form the **vasculature** and **skeletal** components of the lower limb.

B. Mesoderm from the somites
 – also migrates into the limb bud and condenses to eventually form the **musculature** components of the lower limb.

C. Future limb mesodermal cells
 – express the homeobox gene **Hox 3.3** before there is any hint of limb bud formation.

D. Limb mesoderm
 – signals ectoderm at the tip of the limb bud to thicken and form the **apical ectodermal ridge (AER)**.

E. Apical ectodermal ridge
 – interacts with underlying mesoderm to promote outgrowth of the limb bud by promoting mitosis and preventing terminal differentiation of mesodermal cells at the tip of the limb bud.

F. Zone of polarizing activity (ZPA)
 – consists of mesodermal cells located at the base of the limb bud.
 – directs the organization of the limb bud and patterning of the digits, both of which involve **retinoic acid (vitamin A)** and homeobox gene **Hox-4**.

G. Digit formation
 – occurs as a result of selected **apoptosis** within the AER such that five separate regions of AER remain at the tips of the future digits.

II. Vasculature (Figure 20-1)

A. Umbilical artery

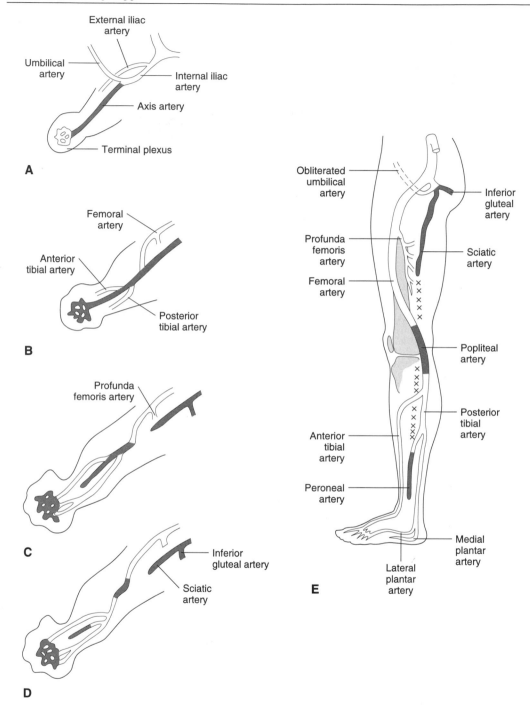

Figure 20-1. Diagram depicting the development of arteries of the lower limb. *(A, B, C, D)* Early limb bud. The earliest arterial supply of the lower limb bud is the axis artery *(dark shading)* and terminal plexus *(dark shading)*, which arise from the umbilical artery. The axis artery gives off branches forming the anterior tibial artery and posterior tibial artery and undergoes regression and some remodeling in selected areas. The external iliac artery gives rise to the femoral artery, which constitutes a separate second arterial channel in the lower limb. *(E)* Adult lower limb. The axis artery persists as the inferior gluteal artery, sciatic artery, proximal part of the popliteal artery, and distal part of the peroneal artery. The *X*'s indicate areas of regression. Bones *(light shading)*.

– gives rise to the **axis artery** of the lower limb, which ends in a **terminal plexus** near the tip of the limb bud.

B. Terminal plexus
– participates in the formation of the **deep plantar arch**.

C. Axis artery
– gives off branches forming the **anterior tibial artery** (which continues as the **dorsalis pedis artery**) and **posterior tibial artery** (which terminates as the **medial plantar artery** and **lateral plantar artery**).
– While most of the axis artery regresses, the axis artery ultimately persists in the adult as the **inferior gluteal artery, sciatic artery** (accompanying the sciatic nerve), proximal part of the **popliteal artery**, and distal part of the **peroneal artery.**

D. External iliac artery
– gives rise to the **femoral artery** of the lower limb, which constitutes a separate second arterial channel into the lower limb that connects to the axis artery.
– The femoral artery gives off the **profunda femoris artery.**

III. Skeletal (Figure 20-2)

A. Lateral plate mesoderm
forms the ilium, ischium, pubis, femur, tibia, fibula, tarsals, metatarsals, and phalanges

B. All bones of the lower limb undergo endochondral ossification

C. Timing of bone formation

1. Week 5: Lateral plate mesoderm within the limb bud condenses

2. Week 6: Condensed mesoderm chondrifies to form a hyaline cartilage model of all lower limb bones

3. Week 7: Primary ossification centers seen in the femur and tibia

4. Week 9 to birth: Primary ossification centers seen in the ilium, ischium, pubis, fibula, calcaneus, talus, metatarsals, and phalanges
   – The ossification of the calcaneus (weeks 16–20) is used medicolegally to establish maturity.

5. Childhood: Secondary ossification centers form in the epiphyseal ends
   – The remaining tarsal bones begin ossification.

IV. Musculature (Figure 20-3 and 20-4)

A. Lower limb bud

1. Lies opposite somites L1, L2, L3, L4, L5, S1, and S2

2. During week 5, mesoderm from these somites (myotomes) migrates into the limb bud and forms a **posterior condensation** and an **anterior condensation**

Week 5

Week 6

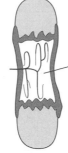

Primary
ossification
center

Weeks 7–9

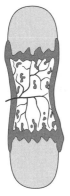

At birth

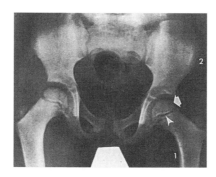

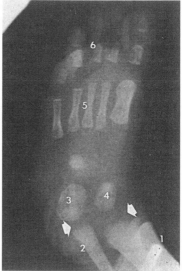

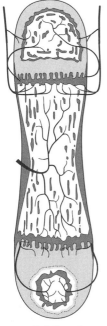

Childhood

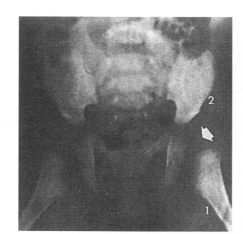

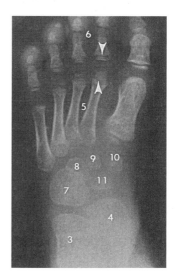

a. The mesoderm of these condensations differentiates into myoblasts; then the condensations split into anatomically recognizable muscles of the lower limb, although little is known about this process

b. Posterior condensation gives rise to these specific muscles: gluteus maximus, gluteus medius, gluteus minimus, piriformis, pectineus, iliacus, tensor fasciae latae, sartorius, rectus femoris, vastus lateralis, vastus medialis, vastus intermedius, short head of biceps femoris, tibialis anterior, extensor hallucis longus, extensor digitorum longus, peroneus tertius, peroneus longus, peroneus brevis, extensor digitorum brevis, extensor hallucis brevis; in general, the **extensor** and **abductor** musculature.

c. Anterior condensation gives rise to these specific muscles: adductor longus, adductor brevis, adductor magnus, gracilis, obturator externus, obturator internus, superior and inferior gemelli, quadratus femoris, semitendinosus, semimembranosus, long head of biceps femoris, gastrocnemius, soleus, plantaris, popliteus, flexor hallucis longus, flexor digitorum longus, tibialis posterior, abductor hallucis, flexor digitorum brevis, abductor digiti minimi, quadratus plantae, lumbricals, flexor hallucis brevis, adductor hallucis, flexor digiti minimi brevis, dorsal and plantar interossei; in general, the **flexor** and **adductor** musculature.

V. Nerves (Lumbosacral Plexus) (see Figure 19-3)

A. Early nerve fibers

– are guided into the limb bud by local cell biological messages at its base; the muscles themselves do not provide any specific target messages to the ingrowing nerve fibers.

Figure 20-2. Bone formation in the lower limb. **Week 5.** Lateral plate mesoderm condenses (*hatched*). **Week 6.** Hyaline cartilage (*light shading*) model of future bones forms. **Weeks 7 to 9.** Primary ossification centers within the diaphysis appear such that bone (*darker shading*) forms (osteogenesis).
At birth: The diaphysis consists of bone (*darker shading*), whereas the epiphysis remains hyaline cartilage (*light shading*). This is important to note when interpreting radiographs of newborns. The radiograph of a newborn at the hip region (*1* = femur; *2* = ilium) shows the portions of the hyaline cartilage model that have been replaced by radiodense bone (*white areas*). Note the epiphyseal end of the femur (*white arrow*) is still hyaline cartilage at birth and therefore will appear radiolucent (*dark area*). The radiograph of a newborn at the ankle and foot shows the portions of the hyaline cartilage model that have been replaced by radiodense bone (*white areas*) in the tibia (*1*), fibula (*2*), calcaneus (*3*), talus (*4*), metatarsals (*5*), and phalanges (*6*). Note that the epiphyseal ends of the tibia and fibula are still cartilage and therefore radiolucent (*white arrows*).
Childhood: During childhood, secondary ossification centers form in the epiphyseal ends of the bones. During childhood and adolescence, the growth in length of long bones occurs at the epiphyseal growth plate. Note the radiograph of a 6-year-old child at the hip region (*1* = femur; *2* = ilium). Since secondary ossification centers are present within the epiphyseal ends, the head of the femur is now radiodense (*white arrow*) and the epiphyseal growth plate (*arrowhead*) where hyaline cartilage is present remains radiolucent (*dark*). This is not to be confused with a bone fracture. On the radiograph of a 6-year-old child at the foot, the diaphyseal and epiphyseal portions of the metatarsals (*5*) and the phalanges (*6*) as well as their epiphyseal growth plates (*arrowheads*) can be observed. The remaining tarsal bones have begun to ossify (*7* = cuboid; *8* = lateral cuneiform; *9* = intermediate cuneiform; *10* = medial cuneiform; *11* = navicular). *3* = calcaneus; *4* = talus. (Radiographs reprinted from Keats TE, Smith TH: *An Atlas of Normal Developmental Roentgen Anatomy*, 2nd ed. Chicago, Year Book Medical Publishers, 1977, pp 31, 237, and 289.)

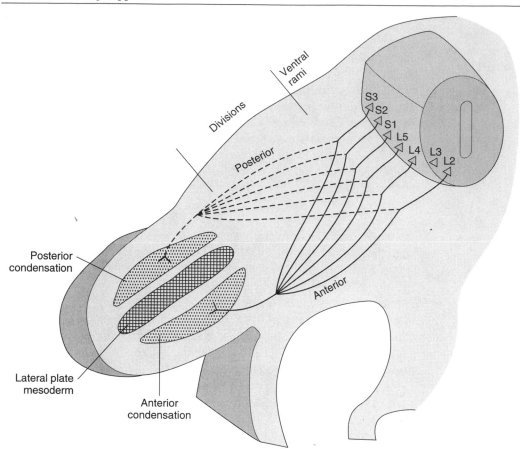

Figure 20-3. Diagram of the muscle and nerve development of the lower limb. Lateral plate mesoderm *(hatched area)* forms down the central axis of the limb bud and is responsible for the formation of the blood vessels and bones of the lower limb. Mesoderm from somites (myotomes) migrates into the limb bud and forms a posterior and anterior condensation *(dotted areas).* Ventral primary rami from L2 to S3 leave the neural tube and divide into posterior *(dotted lines)* and anterior *(solid lines)* divisions. The posterior divisions selectively grow into the posterior condensation. The anterior divisions selectively grow into the anterior condensation.

B. Ventral primary rami from L2, L3, L4, L5, S1, S2, and S3

1. Arrive at the base of the limb bud and divide into **posterior divisions** and **anterior divisions**

   a. Posterior divisions grow into the posterior condensation of mesoderm

      – With further development of the limb musculature, the posterior divisions will form the **superior gluteal nerve (L4, L5, S1), inferior gluteal nerve (L5, S1, S2), femoral nerve (L2, L3, L4), and common peroneal nerve (L4, L5, S1, S2)**, thereby innervating all the muscles that form from the posterior condensation.

   b. Anterior divisions grow into the anterior condensation of mesoderm

      – With further development of the limb musculature, the anterior divisions will form the **tibial nerve (L4, L5, S1, S2, S3)** and **obturator nerve (L2, L3, L4)** and thereby innervate all the muscles that form from the anterior condensation.

VI. Rotation (Figure 20-4)

A. Lower limb buds

- appear in week 4 (about 4 days after the upper limb bud) as small bulges oriented in a **coronal plane**.
- undergo a horizontal flexion in week 6 so that they are now oriented in a **parasagittal plane**.

B. Lower limbs

- rotate medially 90° during weeks 6 to 8 such that the knee points anteriorly, the extensor compartment lies anterior, and the flexor compartment lies posterior.
- This rotation causes the originally straight segmental pattern of innervation (dermatomes) to be somewhat modified in the adult.
- Note that the upper limbs rotate laterally 90°, whereas the lower limbs rotate medially 90°, which sets up the following anatomic situations:

1. Flexor compartment of upper limb is anterior, whereas flexor compartment of lower limb is posterior

2. Extensor compartment of upper limb is posterior, whereas extensor compartment of lower limb is anterior

3. Flexion at wrist joint is analogous to plantar flexion at ankle joint

4. Extension at wrist joint is analogous to dorsiflexion at ankle joint

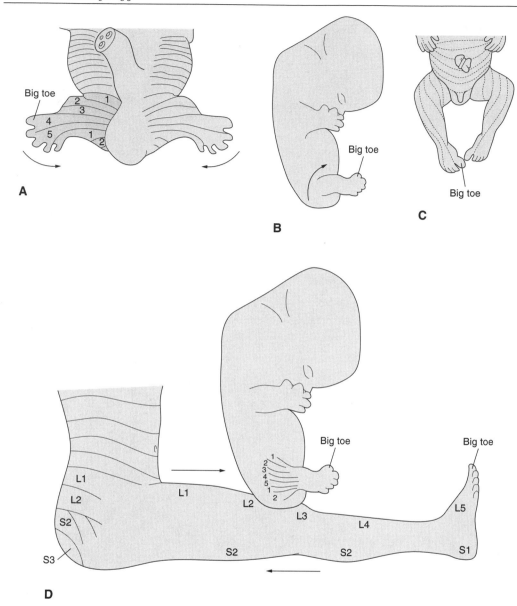

Figure 20-4. Rotation of the lower limb. *(A)* Ventral view of a week 4 embryo. Lower limb buds are oriented in a coronal plane. Note the segmental pattern of innervation from L1 to S2. In week 6, the lower limbs undergo a horizontal flexion *(curved arrows)* such that the lower limb buds become oriented in a parasagittal plane (as shown in *B*). *(B)* Side view of a week 6 embryo. Note the lower limb oriented in a parasagittal plane. During weeks 6 to 8, the lower limb buds rotate 90° medially *(curved arrow)*. *(C)* Ventral view of a week 8 embryo. Note the position of the lower limb with knees pointing anterior. *(D)* Dermatome pattern in the adult lower limb and limb bud. The 90° medial rotation of the lower limb bud causes the originally straight segmental pattern of innervation in the embryo to be somewhat modified ("twisted in a spiral") such that the dermatome pattern in the adult is altered. However, an orderly dermatome pattern can still be recognized in the adult if the lower limb is positioned in a parasagittal plane with the big toe pointing superiorly (as shown). The dermatomes from L1 can be counted distally down the superior border of the lower limb *(arrow)* to L5 and then back proximally up the inferior border of the lower limb *(arrow)* to S2. Note the position of the big toes in *A, B, C,* and *D*. (*A:* Redrawn with permission from Sadler TW: *Langman's Medical Embryology,* 7th ed. Baltimore, Williams & Wilkins, 1996, p 170. *C:* Redrawn with permission from Larson WJ: *Human Embryology,* 2nd ed. New York, Churchill Livingstone, 1997, p 323.)

Review Test

Directions: Each of the numbered items or incomplete statements in this section is followed by answers or by completions of the statement. Select the **one** lettered answer or completion that is **best** in each case.

1. Which of the following arteries gives rise to the axis artery of the lower limb?

(A) external iliac artery
(B) femoral artery
(C) profunda femoris artery
(D) umbilical artery
(E) inferior gluteal artery

2. The femur develops from which of the following?

(A) somite mesoderm
(B) lateral plate mesoderm
(C) intermediate mesoderm
(D) extraembryonic mesoderm
(E) sclerotome mesoderm

3. The rectus femoris muscle develops from which of the following?

(A) posterior condensation
(B) anterior condensation
(C) lateral plate mesoderm
(D) extraembryonic mesoderm
(E) sclerotome mesoderm

4. Which of the following muscles will the posterior divisions of the lumbosacral plexus innervate?

(A) semitendinosus
(B) semimembranosus
(C) long head of biceps femoris
(D) rectus femoris
(E) gastrocnemius

5. During weeks 6 to 8, the lower limb bud will rotate

(A) medially 90°
(B) laterally 90°
(C) medially 180°
(D) laterally 180°
(E) No rotation occurs

Answers and Explanations

1–D. Early in development, the umbilical artery gives rise to the axis artery.

2–B. All bones of the lower limb form from lateral plate mesoderm that condenses along the central axis of the lower limb bud.

3–A. Somite mesoderm migrates into the limb bud and forms two condensations. The posterior condensation of the lower limb gives rise to the extensors of the lower limb, which attain an anterior location in the adult because of the medial rotation of 90°.

4–D. One of the nerves that forms from the posterior divisions of the lumbosacral plexus is the femoral nerve. Posterior divisions of the lumbosacral plexus will innervate muscles derived from the posterior condensation (extensors). Rectus femoris muscle is an extensor at the knee joint. Note that the rectus femoris muscle and the femoral nerve are related embryologically to the posterior condensation and posterior divisions even though in the adult they are located anterior. This occurs because of the medial rotation of 90°.

5–A. The lower limb bud will rotate medially 90° so that the knee points anteriorly.

21

Body Cavities

I. The Intraembryonic Coelom

A. Formation of the intraembryonic coelom (Figure 21-1)

- Formation of the intraembryonic coelom begins when spaces coalesce within the lateral mesoderm and form a horseshoe-shaped space that opens into the chorionic cavity (extraembryonic coelom) on the right and left side.

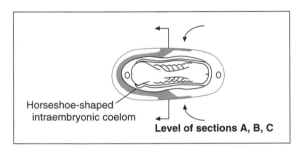

Horseshoe-shaped intraembryonic coelom

Level of sections A, B, C

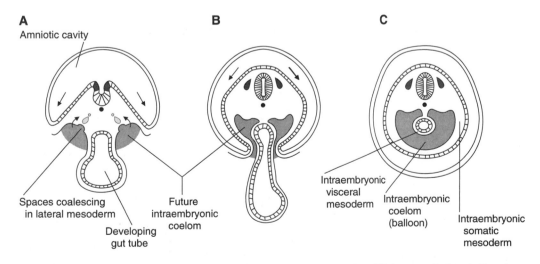

A
Amniotic cavity

B

C

Spaces coalescing in lateral mesoderm

Developing gut tube

Future intraembryonic coelom

Intraembryonic visceral mesoderm

Intraembryonic coelom (balloon)

Intraembryonic somatic mesoderm

Figure 21-1. Diagram illustrating the formation of the intraembryonic coelom (IC) in an early (week 4) embryo. Figure in upper left is a top view showing the horseshoe-shaped IC *(shaded)*. The *curved arrows* indicate the two openings into the chorionic cavity (extraembryonic coelom) on the right and left side. *(A, B, C)* Cross sections showing various stages of IC formation while the embryo undergoes lateral folding.

- The intraembryonic coelom is remodeled due to the craniocaudal folding and lateral folding of the embryo.
- The intraembryonic coelom can best be visualized as a **balloon** whose walls are visceral mesoderm (closest to the viscera) and somatic mesoderm (closest to the body wall).
- provides the needed room for growth of various organs.

B. Partitioning of the intraembryonic coelom

- The intraembryonic coelom is initially one continuous space; to form the definitive adult **pericardial, pleural,** and **peritoneal cavities,** two partitions must develop.
- The two partitions are the **paired pleuropericardial membranes** and the **diaphragm.**

1. Paired pleuropericardial membranes (Figure 21-2)

- are sheets of somatic mesoderm that separate the **pericardial cavity** from the **pleural cavities.**
- Formation appears to be aided by lung buds invading the lateral body wall and by tension on the common cardinal veins resulting from rapid longitudinal growth.
- develop into the definitive **fibrous pericardium** surrounding the heart.

2. Diaphragm (Figure 21-3)

- separates the **pleural cavities** from the **peritoneal cavity.**
- is formed through the fusion of tissue from four different sources:

a. Septum transversum

- is a thick mass of mesoderm located between the primitive heart tube and the developing liver.
- is the primordium of the **central tendon of the diaphragm** in the adult.

b. Paired pleuroperitoneal membranes

- are sheets of somatic mesoderm.

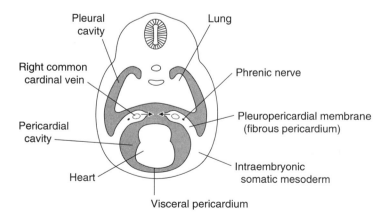

Figure 21-2. Cross section showing two folds of intraembryonic somatic mesoderm carrying the phrenic nerves and common cardinal veins. The two folds fuse in the midline *(arrows)* to form the pleuropericardial membrane. This separates the pericardial cavity *(shaded)* from the pleural cavity *(shaded).*

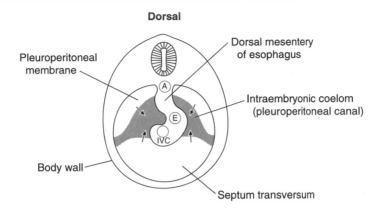

Figure 21-3. Cross section of an embryo at week 5 showing the four components that fuse *(arrows)* to form the diaphragm, which closes off the intraembryonic coelom between the pleural and peritoneal cavities. The portions of the intraembryonic coelom that connect the pleural and pericardial cavities in the embryo are called the pleuroperitoneal canals *(shaded).* A = aorta; E = esophagus; *IVC* = Inferior vena cava.

- appear to develop from the dorsal and dorsolateral body wall by an unknown mechanism.

c. Dorsal mesentery of the esophagus

- Myoblasts invade this mesentery to form the **crura of the diaphragm** in the adult.

d. Body wall

- contributes muscle to the peripheral portions of the definitive diaphragm.

II. Positional Changes of the Diaphragm

- During week 4 of development, the developing diaphragm becomes innervated by the **phrenic nerves**, which originate from **C3, C4, and C5** and pass through the pleuropericardial membranes (this explains the definitive location of the phrenic nerves associated with the **fibrous pericardium**).
- By week 8, there is an apparent **descent of the diaphragm to L1** because of the rapid growth of the neural tube.
- The phrenic nerves are carried along with the "descending diaphragm," which explains their unusually long length in the adult.

III. Clinical Considerations

A. Congenital diaphragmatic hernia

- is a herniation of abdominal contents into the pleural cavity.
- is caused by a **failure of the pleuroperitoneal membrane** to develop or fuse with the other components of the diaphragm.
- is most commonly found on the **left posterolateral side**.
- is usually life-threatening because abdominal contents compress the lung buds, causing **pulmonary hypoplasia**.
- Clinical signs in the newborn are an **unusually flat abdomen, breathlessness,** and **cyanosis**.
- can be detected prenatally using ultrasonography.

B. **Esophageal hiatal hernia**
   - is a herniation of the stomach through the esophageal hiatus into the pleural cavity.
   - is caused by an abnormally large esophageal hiatus.
   - renders the **esophagogastric sphincter** incompetent so that stomach contents reflux into the esophagus.
   - Clinical signs in the newborn are **vomiting (frequently projectile) when the infant is laid on its back after feeding**.

Review Test

Directions: Each of the numbered items or incomplete statements in this section is followed by answers or by completions of the statement. Select the **one** lettered answer or completion that is **best** in each case.

1. A congenital diaphragmatic hernia may result from failure of the

(A) septum transversum to develop
(B) pleuroperitoneal membranes to fuse in a normal fashion
(C) pleuropericardial membrane to develop completely
(D) dorsal mesentery of the esophagus to develop
(E) body wall to form the peripheral part of the diaphragm

2. A congenital diaphragmatic hernia most commonly occurs

(A) on the right anteromedial side
(B) on the right posterolateral side
(C) on the left anteromedial side
(D) on the left posterolateral side
(E) anywhere on the left side

3. A congenital diaphragmatic hernia is usually life-threatening because it is associated with

(A) pulmonary hypoplasia
(B) pulmonary hyperplasia
(C) physiologic umbilical hernia
(D) liver hypoplasia
(E) liver agenesis

4. An 8-day-old boy presents with a history of complete loss of breath at times and of turning blue on a number of occasions. If the baby is placed in an upright or sitting position, his breathing improves. Physical examination reveals an unusually flat stomach when the newborn is lying down; auscultation demonstrates no breath sounds on the left side of the thorax. What is the diagnosis?

(A) Physiologic umbilical herniation
(B) Esophageal hiatal hernia
(C) Tetralogy of Fallot
(D) Congenital diaphragmatic hernia
(E) Tricuspid atresia

5. During week 4, the developing diaphragm is located at

(A) C3, C4, C5
(B) T3, T4, T5
(C) T8, T9, T10
(D) L1, L2, L3
(E) L4, L5, L6

6. An apparently healthy newborn with a hearty appetite has begun feedings with formula. When she is laid down in the crib after feeding, she experiences projectile vomiting. Which of the following conditions is a probable cause of this vomiting?

(A) Physiologic umbilical herniation
(B) Esophageal hiatal hernia
(C) Tetralogy of Fallot
(D) Congenital diaphragmatic hernia
(E) Tracheoesophageal fistula

Directions: The numbered items below correspond to lettered items in the figure. For each numbered item, select the **one** lettered option that is most closely associated with it. Each lettered option may be selected once, more than once, or not at all.

Questions 7–13

For each statement concerning the developing diaphragm, select the most appropriate structure in the diagram.

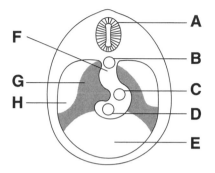

7. Forms the central tendon of the diaphragm

8. Its abnormal development or fusion causes congenital diaphragmatic hernia

9. Forms the crura of the diaphragm

10. Pleuroperitoneal canal

11. Inferior vena cava

12. Esophagus

13. Aorta

Answers and Explanations

1–B. The formation of the diaphragm occurs through the fusion of tissue from four different sources. The pleuroperitoneal membranes normally fuse with the three other components during week 6 of development. Abnormal development or fusion of one or both of the pleuroperitoneal membranes causes a patent opening between the thorax and abdomen through which abdominal viscera may herniate.

2–D. Congenital diaphragmatic hernias occur most commonly on the left posterolateral side. The pleuroperitoneal membrane on the right side closes before the left for reasons that are not clear. Consequently, the patency on the left side remains unclosed for a longer time. The portion of the diaphragm formed by the pleuroperitoneal membrane in the newborn is located posterolateral.

3–A. The herniation of abdominal contents into the pleural cavity compresses the developing lung bud, resulting in pulmonary hypoplasia. Lung development on the ipsilateral (left) side of the herniation is most commonly affected, but lung development on the contralateral (right) side can also be compromised. The lungs may achieve normal size and function after surgical reduction of the hernia and repair of the diaphragm. However, mortality is high due to pulmonary hypoplasia.

4–D. Loss of breath and cyanosis result from pulmonary hypoplasia associated with congenital diaphragmatic hernia. Placing the baby in an upright position will reduce the hernia somewhat and ease the pressure on the lungs, thereby increasing the baby's comfort. The baby's stomach is flat (instead of the plump belly of a normal newborn) because the abdominal viscera have herniated into the thorax. Auscultation reveals no breath sounds on the left side because of pulmonary hypoplasia.

5–A. Although it may seem unusual, the adult diaphragm has its embryologic beginning at the cervical level (C3, C4, C5). Nerve roots from C3, C4, and C5 enter the developing diaphragm, bringing both motor and sensory innervation. With the subsequent rapid growth of the neural tube, there is an apparent descent of the diaphragm to its adult levels (thoracic and lumbar). However, the diaphragm retains its innervation from C3, C4, and C5, which explains the unusually long phrenic nerves.

6–B. An esophageal hiatal hernia is a herniation of the stomach through the esophageal hiatus into the pleural cavity. This compromises the esophagogastric sphincter so that stomach contents can easily reflux into the esophagus. The combination of a full stomach after feeding and lying down in the crib will cause vomiting in this newborn.

7–E. The septum transversum forms the central tendon of the diaphragm in the adult.

8–H. The pleuroperitoneal membranes located in a posterolateral position are a factor in congenital diaphragmatic hernia, especially on the left side.

9–F. Myoblasts will invade the dorsal mesentery of the esophagus, forming the crura of the diaphragm.

10–G. The pleuroperitoneal canal is a part of the intraembryonic coelom that connects the pleural and peritoneal cavities. In normal development, it gets closed due to the formation of the diaphragm. If it remains open, a congenital diaphragmatic hernia occurs.

11–D. The inferior vena cava penetrates the diaphragm en route to the right atrium. Embryologically, the inferior vena cava is found in the dorsal mesentery of the esophagus in a most ventral position.

12–C. The esophagus penetrates the diaphragm en route to the stomach. Embryologically, it is suspended from the dorsal mesentery of the esophagus, which forms part of the diaphragm. The esophagus is located in a central position between the dorsal aorta and ventral inferior vena cava.

13–B. The aorta penetrates the diaphragm. Embryologically, the aorta is found in the dorsal mesentery of the esophagus in a most dorsal position.

22

Fetal Period (Weeks 9–38)

I. Overview

A. General (Figure 22-1)

- The fetal period (weeks 9–38) is characterized by **rapid body and organ growth**.
- The most striking feature of the fetal period is the relative reduction of head growth compared to body growth.

B. Length of pregnancy

- is computed by adding 280 days (40 weeks) to the onset of the last menstruation, or by adding 266 days (38 weeks) to the date of fertilization. (*Note:* In this book, "fertilization age" is used.)

C. Age determination of the fetus

- Ultrasound measurements predict fetal age with an accuracy of ± 1–2 days.

  1. Crown–rump length (CRL; sitting height)
  - is the length from the vertex to the base of the buttocks.
  - CRL measurement is the usual and most accurate method of determining fetal age.

  2. Crown–heel length (CHL; standing height)
  - is the length from the vertex to the heel.

  3. Foot length
  - correlates well with CRL.

II. Monthly Periods of Fetal Development

- This section includes the developmental events of the third through the ninth months (week 9 through week 38).

A. Third month (weeks 9–12)

1. Head size is about half of CRL.

2. Intestines are found in the umbilical cord and then return to the abdominal cavity.

3. Eyelids grow together and fuse.

245

Growth in Length and Weight During the Fetal Period

Age (weeks)	Age (months)	CRL (cm)	Weight (g)
9–12	3rd	5–8	10–45
13–16	4th	9–14	60–200
17–20	5th	15–19	250–450
21–24	6th	20–23	500–820
25–28	7th	24–27	900–1300
29–32	8th	28–30	1400–2100
33–38	9th	31–36	2200–3400

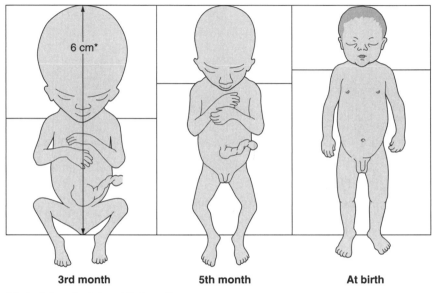

3rd month	**5th month**	**At birth**

* Actual size of a fetus at 3rd month

Figure 22-1. Growth in length and weight during the fetal period. *CRL* = crown–rump length. (Modified from Sadler TW: *Langman's Medical Embryology,* 7th ed. Baltimore, Williams & Wilkins, pp 91–92.)

4. Lanugo (fine hair) appears.

5. Primary ossification centers appear in the long bones and skull.

6. Kidneys secrete **urine** into the amniotic fluid.

7. Male and female external genitalia can be recognized.

8. Liver is an important site of **hemopoiesis**.

B. Fourth month (weeks 13–16)

1. Ossification of the skeleton is extensive.

2. Body hair starts developing.

3. Spleen is an important site of **hemopoiesis**.

4. Eyes, ears, and nose approach typical appearance.

5. Eye movements begin.

6. Ovaries contain **primordial follicles**.

7. Coordinated limb movements occur but cannot be detected by the mother.

8. **Bile** is secreted into the duodenum.

9. **Meconium** (epithelial cells, mucus, and bile) is found in the gastrointestinal tract.

C. Fifth month (weeks 17–20)

1. Coordinated limb movements occur and can be detected by the mother as **quickening**; parturition follows quickening by approximately 147 days.

2. **Lanugo** and **vernix caseosa** (a mixture of sebum, epidermal cells, and lanugo) cover the skin; vernix caseosa protects the skin from maceration by the amniotic fluid.

3. Eyebrows and head hair appear at end of this period.

4. **Brown fat** accumulates in the neck and perirenal areas of the fetus; it has a rich blood supply and plays a role in the **regulation of fetal body temperature**.

5. The uterus forms.

6. The testes form and begin their descent into the scrotum.

7. **Fetal heartbeat** can be heard with a stethoscope.

D. Sixth month (weeks 21–24)

1. Rapid eye movements begin.

2. Skin is wrinkled and pink or red.

3. **Blink–startle reflex** is demonstrable on vibroacoustic stimulation of mother's abdomen.

4. Fingernails are present.

5. **Surfactant** is secreted by **Type II pneumocytes** of the lungs.

E. Seventh month (weeks 25–28)

1. Eyelids separate.

2. Hair is present on the head.

3. **Lungs are capable of breathing air;** respiratory bronchioles are formed.

F. Eighth month (weeks 29–32)

1. Toenails are present

2. Fingernails reach fingertips.

3. **Pupillary light reflex** is present.

4. Testes are descending.

5. Skin is pink and smooth.

G. Ninth month (weeks 33–38)

1. Toenails reach toetips

2. Fingernails extend beyond fingertips.

3. Lanugo hairs are almost absent.

4. Testes are in scrotum.

5. Fetus has firm hand grip and orients to light.

6. Head size is one-fourth of CRL.

7. **Bone marrow** is an important site of **hemopoiesis**.

8. At term (38 weeks), the fetus has a CRL of 36 cm and a weight of 3400 g.

9. At term (38 weeks), brain weight is 350 g whereas brain weight is 1400 g in the adult.

III. Factors Affecting Fetal Growth

A. Retarded growth

1. **Maternal malnutrition**
   - is the most common cause of **intrauterine growth retardation (IUGR)**.

2. **Substance abuse**
   - **Alcohol abuse and cigarette smoking** both result in IUGR (see Chapter 23).
   - **Marijuana (cannabis), heroin,** and **methadone** are reported to cause IUGR.

3. **Impaired uteroplacental blood flow**
   - results from hypoplastic chorionic or umbilical vessels and renal disease.
   - may result in fetal starvation.

4. **Placental insufficiency**
   - results from placental infarction and is found in some degree in more than 50% of placentas examined at birth; results in **placental dysfunction syndrome**.
   - is the most common cause of very low birth weight in full-term fetuses.

5. **Genetic factors**
   - **Trisomy 21 (Down syndrome)** and **trisomy 18 (Edwards' syndrome)** result in retarded fetal growth.

B. Excessive growth
- **Maternal diabetes** may result in larger than normal babies, with hyperplasia of the pancreatic islets of Langerhans.
- Abortions, stillbirths, and neonatal death rates are higher in diabetic mothers than in nondiabetic mothers.

IV. Viruses That Affect the Fetus

A. Rubella

– Infection in the fetal period may damage the central nervous system (CNS), the eye, and the ear.

B. Cytomegalovirus (CMV)

– is the most common virus affecting the human fetus.
– may damage the CNS, the eye, and the ear.

V. Viability of the Fetus

– Fetuses born younger than 20 weeks' gestation rarely survive.
– Fetuses born weighing less than 500 g rarely survive.
– Fetuses born between week 25 and 28 have functional lungs and can survive with intensive care.
– Most prenatal deaths occur in fetuses younger than week 32 and less than 2000 g in weight.

VI. Prenatal Diagnostic Procedures

A. Amniocentesis

– is the **aspiration of fluid** from the amniotic sac.
– is performed between weeks 12 and 14.
– has a 0.5% risk of miscarriage.
– is used to perform the following studies:

1. Alpha-fetoprotein assay

– is used to diagnose **neural tube defects**, such as spina bifida or anencephaly.

2. Spectrophotometry

– is used to diagnose **hemolytic disease of the newborn** (erythroblastosis fetalis) due to Rh-incompatibility.

3. Sex chromatin studies

– are used to determine fetal sex.
– are used to diagnose sex-linked hereditary diseases, such as X-linked recessive **muscular dystrophy (Duchenne)** and **hemophilia**.

4. Cell culture studies

– are used to diagnose **chromosomal anomalies**, such as trisomy 21, and **enzyme deficiencies**.

5. Enzyme analysis (Table 22-1)

6. DNA analysis (Tables 22-2 and 22-3)

– **Southern blotting** is a technique of DNA analysis used to identify defective chromosomes early in pregnancy; a useful technique in genetic counseling.

B. Chorionic villus biopsy

– is used for chromosomal studies and to diagnose enzyme deficiencies.
– may be performed in week 7, a major advantage over amniocentesis.
– has a 1% risk of miscarriage.

– Tissue may be directly karyotyped, or karyotyped after culture.
– yields larger cell samples than amniocentesis.
– is used for **Southern blotting**.

C. Cordocentesis

– is a technique used to sample **fetal blood** directly from the umbilical cord.
– is used for quick chromosome analysis (karyotyping) or hematologic studies.

D. Tests using maternal serum

1. Maternal serum alpha-fetoprotein (MSAFP) assay

– is used to diagnose **neural tube defects** (spina bifida); MSAFP is elevated.
– is used to screen for **Down syndrome**; MSAFP is reduced.

Table 22-1. Metabolic Disorders That can be Diagnosed by Enzyme Analysis in Cells Cultured from Chorionic Villi or Amniotic Fluid

Carbohydrate disorders Galactosemia Glycogen storage disease	**Lysosomal storage diseases** Gangliosidosis 1 Gangliosidosis 2 (Tay-Sachs disease)
Aminoacidopathies Maple syrup urine disease	**Disorders of hormone synthesis** Steroid sulfatase deficiency
Organic acidemias Methylmalonic acidemia	**Disorders of connective tissue** Hypophosphatasia
Purine and pyrimidine disorders Adenosine deaminase deficiency	

Modified from Thompson MW, McInnes RR, Willard HF: *Genetics in Medicine*, 5th ed. Philadelphia, WB Saunders, 1991, p 420.

Table 22-2. Some Single-Gene Disorders That can be Diagnosed Prenatally by DNA Analysis

Cystic fibrosis (AR)*

Hematologic disease
Hemophilia A and B (X-linked)
Sickle cell anemia (AR)
Thalassemia α and β (AR)

Neurologic disease
Huntington's disease (AD)†
Muscular dystrophy (Duchenne and Becker) [X-linked]
Myotonic dystrophy (AD)
Neurofibromatosis type I (AD)
Retinoblastoma (AD)
Tay-Sachs disease [GM_2 gangliosidosis] (AR)

Phenylketonuria (AR)

*Autosomal recessive; †autosomal dominant.
Modified from Thompson MW, McInnes RR, Willard HF: *Genetics in Medicine*, 5th ed. Philadelphia, WB Saunders, 1991, p 413.

Table 22-3. Prenatal Diagnosis by DNA Analysis

Test	Disorders Diagnosed
Direct Methods	
Southern blotting to detect gene deletions or rearrangements	Duchenne muscular dystrophy (60% of mutations that cause it are deletions)
Southern blotting and restriction enzyme analysis to detect point mutations that alter restriction sites	Sickle cell anemia and hemophilia A
Allele-specific oligonucleotides to detect previously characterized mutations	Cystic fibrosis
Polymerase chain reaction amplification to detect deletions or previously characterized mutations	Duchenne muscle dystrophy, Lesch-Nyhan syndrome, Tay-Sachs disease, and cystic fibrosis
Indirect Method	
DNA polymorphisms within or near disease loci to detect mutations in a particular gene	Phenylketonuria and hemophilia A

Modified from Thompson MW, McInnes RR, Willard HF: *Genetics in Medicine*, 5th ed. Philadelphia, WB Saunders, 1991, p 420.

2. Unconjugated estriol

– is reduced in Down syndrome and in cases of fetal immaturity.

3. Human chorionic gonadotropin (hCG)

– is significantly higher in Down syndrome.

E. Ultrasonography (Table 22-4)

– is used to monitor needle and catheter insertion for amniocentesis and chorionic villus biopsy.
– has no known contraindications.
– is used for fetal sex determination as early as week 12.
– is used to measure placental and fetal size, to diagnose abnormal presentations, and to diagnose fetal malformations (neural tube defects, hydrocephalus, and microcephalus) prenatally.

Table 22-4. Congenital Anomalies That can be Diagnosed Prenatally by Ultrasonography

Single-gene disorders
Polycystic kidney disease
Skeletal dysplasias (achondroplasia)
Multifactorial disorders
Cleft lip and palate
Congenital heart defects (tetralogy of Fallot)
Neural tube defects (spina bifida)

Modified from Thompson MW, McInnes RR, Willard HF: *Genetics in Medicine*, 5th ed. Philadelphia, WB Saunders, 1991, p 418.

Review Test

Directions: Each of the numbered items or incomplete statements in this section is followed by answers or by completions of the statement. Select the **one** lettered answer or completion that is **best** in each case.

1. All of the following statements concerning the fetal period are true EXCEPT

(A) the fetus is less sensitive to teratogenic agents than the embryo
(B) most organ systems have developed before the fetal period
(C) the CNS continues its development throughout the fetal period
(D) during fetal growth the head becomes proportionally larger than the body
(E) the fetal period extends from week 9 of development to birth

2. Fetal age is usually and most accurately estimated by

(A) biparietal diameter (BPD) of the head
(B) cheek-to-cheek width
(C) crown-heel length (CHL)
(D) crown-rump length (CRL)
(E) foot length

3. Which of the following gestational weeks is the earliest date at which the sex of a fetus can be determined by examination of the external genitalia?

(A) Week 8
(B) Week 10
(C) Week 12
(D) Week 14
(E) Week 16

4. All of the following events happen in the gestational weeks 9 through 12 EXCEPT

(A) lanugo appears
(B) primary ossification centers appear
(C) coordinated limb movements occur
(D) eyelids fuse
(E) fetus doubles its CRL

5. All of the following statements concerning vernix caseosa are correct EXCEPT

(A) it contains sebum
(B) it contains epidermal cells
(C) it contains lanugo
(D) it contains decidual cells
(E) it protects the skin from maceration

6. Quickening is first observed by the mother in which gestational period?

(A) Weeks 9–12
(B) Weeks 13–16
(C) Weeks 17–20
(D) Weeks 21–24
(E) Weeks 22–28

7. All of the following are signs of a viable fetus EXCEPT

(A) weighs 500 g
(B) fingernails reach fingertips
(C) toenails present
(D) CRL measures 35 cm
(E) testes in scrotum

8. The major advantage of chorionic villus biopsy (CVB) over amniocentesis is

(A) CVB can be used to detect chromosomal abnormalities
(B) CVB can be used to detect inborn errors of metabolism
(C) CVB can be performed at week 7 of development
(D) CVB can be used to detect X-linked disorders
(E) CVB can be used to detect neural tube defects

9. Each of the following statements concerning amniocentesis is true EXCEPT

(A) it is used to detect neural tube defects
(B) it is used to detect alpha-fetoprotein
(C) it is used to detect Down syndrome
(D) it is used to detect erythroblastosis fetalis
(E) it can be performed in the seventh week after fertilization

10. Very low birth weight in a full-term fetus would most likely result from

(A) heavy cigarette smoking
(B) alcohol abuse
(C) maternal diabetes
(D) placental insufficiency
(E) maternal malnutrition

11. Each of the following statements concerning brown fat is correct EXCEPT

(A) it is a site of heat production
(B) it is found in the neck and around the kidneys
(C) it first appears in week 9
(D) it is multilocular adipose tissue
(E) its adipocytes contain numerous mitochondria

12. Surfactant is produced by

(A) Type I pneumocytes
(B) Type II pneumocytes
(C) endothelial cells
(D) macrophages
(E) squamous alveolar cells

Directions: Each group of items in this section consists of lettered options followed by a set of numbered items. For each item, select the **one** lettered option that is most closely associated with it. Each lettered option may be selected once, more than once, or not at all.

Questions 13–20

Match each of the following developments with the fetal period in which it occurs.

(A) Weeks 9–12
(B) Weeks 13–16
(C) Weeks 17–20
(D) Weeks 21–24
(E) Weeks 25–28
(F) Weeks 29–32
(G) Weeks 33–38

13. Head is half of CRL

14. Brain weighs 350 g

15. Pupillary light reflex present

16. Sex can be determined by ultrasound examination

17. Heartbeat audible with stethoscope

18. Skeleton clearly visible on x-ray

19. Skin wrinkled and red

20. Quickening and brown fat

Directions: Each group of items in this section consists of lettered options followed by a set of numbered items. For each item, select the **one** lettered option that is most closely associated with it. Each lettered option may be selected once, more than once, or not at all.

Questions 21–27

For each of the following characteristics, choose the appropriate prenatal test.

(A) Amniocentesis
(B) Chorionic villus biopsy
(C) Cordocentesis
(D) Maternal serum alpha-fetoprotein assay
(E) Southern blotting
(F) Ultrasonography

21. Could be used to diagnose microcephaly

22. Is a technique used to sample fetal blood for karyotyping

23. May be performed in week 7

24. Has a 0.5% risk factor for abortion

25. Has a 1% risk factor for abortion

26. Is a technique of DNA analysis that is used to identify defective chromosomes early in pregnancy

27. Is usually performed between weeks 12 and 14

Answers and Explanations

1–D. During the fetal period the head becomes proportionally smaller than the body. At week 9, the head is half of the crown–rump length (CRL); at week 38, the head is one-quarter of the CRL.

2–D. Fetal age is usually and most accurately estimated by crown–rump length (CRL). Foot length correlates well with CRL and is used to estimate the age of an incomplete fetus. Fetal head measurements are especially important in women who have a narrow pelvis.

3–C. The sex of a fetus can be determined by examination of the external genitalia during week 12. From weeks 1 to 6 the male and female external genitalia are indifferent (indifferent embryo). By week 20, phenotypic differentiation of external genitalia is complete.

4–C. Coordinated limb movements occur in the fourth month (weeks 13–16); these movements cannot be detected by the mother. The first random movements of the extremities occur in week 8. Distinct movements of the limbs (quickening) are felt by the mother in the fifth month (weeks 17–20). Parturition is reported to occur 147 ± 15 days after quickening.

5–D. Vernix caseosa covers and protects the fetal skin from maceration by the amniotic fluid. It consists of sebum (secretion of the sebaceous glands), epidermal cells, and lanugo. Decidual cells make up the functional layer of the endometrium; they are not found in the amniotic sac.

6–C. Quickening (fetal movements) is first felt by the mother in the fifth month (weeks 17–20).

7–A. Fetuses that weigh less than 500 g rarely survive. Toenails are present and fingernails reach the fingertips in the eighth month (weeks 29–32). At birth, the testes should be in the scrotum or palpable within the inguinal canals. At birth, a crown–rump length (CRL) of 35 cm is normal and equals a crown–heel length (CHL) of 50 cm. Fetuses older than week 30 have a good chance to survive.

8–C. The advantage of chorionic villus biopsy (CVB) over amniocentesis is that CVB can be performed at week 7, whereas amniocentesis is usually performed during weeks 12 to 14.

9–E. Amniocentesis is usually performed during weeks 12 to 14 because 25 ml of amniotic fluid is needed for analysis in amniocentesis; this volume is not available before week 12. Amniocentesis is used to detect alpha-fetoprotein, levels of which are elevated when the fetus has a neural tube defect. Amniocentesis is used in detecting hemolytic disease of the newborn and chromosomal abnormalities, such as Down syndrome.

10–D. Placental insufficiency is the most common cause of very low birth weight (less than 2500 g; average birth weight is 3400 g). Placental insufficiency usually results from infarction of the placenta, resulting in a reduction of nutrient exchange between the fetal and maternal circulation. Cigarette smoking and maternal malnutrition result in low birth weight. Diabetic mothers produce larger than average infants.

11–C. Brown fat first appears in weeks 17 to 20. Brown fat is multilocular adipose tissue found in the neck and around the kidneys; it plays a role in heat production. The brown color is due to a high density of capillaries and mitochondria.

12–B. Surfactant is elaborated by Type II pneumocytes (great alveolar cells) in the lungs; it is produced by week 24. Insufficient surfactant production results in hyaline membrane disease, the neonatal respiratory disease.

13–A. At week 9, the head is half of the crown-rump length (CRL).

14–G. At birth, the brain weighs 350 g; the adult brain weighs 1400 g. At birth, the brain is 25% of body weight (3400 g). The adult brain is about 2% of body weight.

15–F. The pupillary light reflex is present at week 30.

16–A. The sex of the fetus can be determined by ultrasound examination by week 12.

17–C. At week 18, the fetal heartbeat can be heard with a stethoscope.

18–B. The skeleton is clearly visible on x-ray by week 16. Primary ossification sites appear in the long bones and skull as early as week 13.

19–D. At week 22, the skin of the fetus is wrinkled, translucent, and red in color. The lack of subcutaneous fat results in skin wrinkling; the abundance of capillaries accounts for the red color. At week 24, fingernails appear and Type II pneumocytes are elaborating surfactant.

20–C. In weeks 17 to 20, fetal limb movements (quickening) can be felt by the mother; quickening occurs approximately 5 months (147 days) before delivery. Brown fat accumulates in the neck and perirenal areas; brown fat produces heat by oxidation of fatty acids.

21–F. Ultrasonography is used to detect morphologic anomalies, such as hydrocephalus and microcephaly. It permits determination of fetal age and multiple pregnancies and verifies fetal viability.

22–C. Cordocentesis (percutaneous umbilical cord blood sampling) is a technique used to sample fetal blood for karyotyping. It is used for quick chromosome analysis or hematologic studies.

23–B. Chorionic villus biopsy may be performed in week 7, which is its major advantage over amniocentesis. It is used for chromosomal studies and the diagnosis of enzyme deficiencies.

24–A. Amniocentesis has a 0.5% risk factor for abortion; this is less than the risk factor for chorionic villus biopsy (1%).

25–B. Chorionic villus biopsy carries a 1% risk factor for miscarriage.

26–E. Southern blotting is a technique of DNA analysis used to identify defective chromosomes early in pregnancy; it is a useful technique in genetic counseling.

27–A. Amniocentesis is usually performed between weeks 12 and 14. Before week 12 there is not enough amniotic fluid for assay. Approximately 25 ml of amniotic fluid is aspirated for assay.

23

Human Birth Defects

I. Introduction–Human Birth Defects

- may be caused by **environmental or genetic factors**, or a combination of both (multifactorial).
- are caused by **teratogens**, agents that cause congenital malformations.
- Approximately 3% of liveborn infants have defects at birth; this statistic doubles by the end of the first postnatal year.
- Approximately 20% of infant deaths in the United States result from birth defects.
- are typically described as:

A. Malformations: defects in development of an organ or body region resulting from an abnormality in the **developmental potential** of its precursor

B. Disruptions: defects in development of an organ or body region resulting from a **discruption** of an originally normal developmental process of its precursor

C. Deformations: anomalies in the form, shape, or position of an organ or body region caused by an **extrinsic mechanical factor**

D. Agenesis: the absence of an organ or body region resulting from the **absence of its precursor**

E. Aplasia: the absence of an organ or body region resulting from **failure of development** of its precursor

II. Genetic Factors

- The normal human somatic cell has 46 chromosomes; 22 pairs are autosomes, and two are sex chromosomes.
- The normal male karyotype is expressed as 46,XY; the normal female karyotype is expressed as 46,XX.
- Any deviation from the diploid number of 46 chromosomes is called **aneuploidy**, which is the most common type of chromosome abnormality.

A. Numerical chromosomal abnormalities

- If one additional chromosome is present, the condition is called **trisomy**.

257

– If one chromosome is absent, the condition is called **monosomy**.

– Trisomy and monosomy are most often caused by meiotic **nondisjunction** of chromosomes.

1. **Autosomal abnormalities**

   a. **Trisomy 21 (Down syndrome)**

      – is the most common type of trisomy, with an incidence in the general population of 1:800 births.

      – Frequency increases with advancing maternal age; for example, the frequency in babies born to mothers under 25 is about 1:2000 births; the frequency in mothers over 45 is about 1:25.

      – may affect all parts of the brain.

      – is characterized by signs of mental retardation, microcephaly, microphthalmia, colobomata, cataracts and glaucoma, epicanthic folds, simian crease, congenital heart defects. Incidence of umbilical hernia and duodenal atresia is high.

      – Alzheimer neurofibrillary tangles and plaques are found in the brains of persons over 30 years of age who have Down syndrome.

   b. **Trisomy 18 (Edwards' syndrome)**

      – is much less common than trisomy 21; incidence is 1:8000 births.

      – **Infants usually die soon after birth.**

      – is characterized by signs of mental retardation, congenital heart defects, prominent occiput, low-set ears, micrognathia, flexed digits, and rocker-bottom feet.

   c. **Trisomy 13 (Patau syndrome)**

      – is much less common than either trisomy 21 or trisomy 18, with an incidence of 1:25,000 births.

      – **Infants usually die soon after birth.**

      – is characterized by signs of mental retardation, microphthalmia, congenital heart defects, deafness, colobomata, and cleft lip and cleft palate.

2. **Sex chromosome abnormalities**

   a. **Klinefelter syndrome (47,XXY)**

      – is found **only in males** with an incidence of 1:1000 male births.

      – is characterized by **male hypogonadism**, sterility, and gynecomastia. Males who have Klinefelter syndrome are usually tall and eunuchoid.

      – Some persons with this syndrome have 48 chromosomes (i.e., 44 autosomes and 4 sex chromosomes [48,XXXY]).

      – Various **mosaics** (47,XXY/46,XY) can occur. (A mosaic is an individual who has at least two cell lines differing in genotype or karyotype.)

   b. **XYY syndrome (47,XYY)**: an aneuploidy of the sex chromosomes.

   c. **Turner syndrome (45,XO) [monosomy X chromosome]**

      – is found **only in females**, with an incidence of 1:5000 live female births. Only 1% of embryos survive.

      – is the classic form of **female hypogonadism (gonadal dysgenesis)**.

- Persons with this syndrome have only one single X chromosome and are sex chromatin negative.
- is characterized by such deficits as infantile genitalia, hypoplastic ovaries, congenital heart defects, webbed neck, and lymphedema of the extremities.
- Various mosaics may occur.
- is the most common cause of **primary amenorrhea**.

d. Triple X syndrome (47,XXX)

- has an incidence of 1:960 births.
- is characterized by the presence of two sex chromatin bodies **(Barr bodies)**.
- Persons with this syndrome are normal in habitus and are usually fertile; 20% are mildly mentally retarded.

B. Structural abnormalities

- result from breakage of chromosomes or faulty repair mechanisms.

1. Cri du chat syndrome

- is classified as a structural **chromosomal abnormality**.
- results from deletion of the short arm of chromosome 5.
- has an incidence of 1:100,000 births.
- is characterized by deficits such as mental retardation, microcephaly, congenital heart defects, and a cat-like cry.

2. Contiguous gene syndromes

- have deletions that affect several contiguous genes (segmental aneusomy).

a. Prader-Willi syndrome

- is associated with deletion of band q12 on **chromosome 15** (found in the **father**).
- is characterized by mental retardation, hyperphagia, and hypogonadism.

b. Angelman syndrome

- is associated with deletion of band q12 on **chromosome 15** (found in the **mother**).
- is characterized by severe mental retardation, seizures, and dystaxia.

c. DiGeorge syndrome

- is associated with deletion of band q11 on **chromosome 22**.
- is characterized by an absence of the thymus and parathyroid glands and T-cell immunodeficiency.

3. Single-gene defect abnormalities

- represent approximately 10% of congenital anomalies.

a. Achondroplasia

- is an autosomal dominant disorder (**dwarfism**) characterized by large head, short stature, short limbs and fingers, and normal trunk.

b. Polydactyly

- is an autosomal dominant disorder characterized by the presence of **extra digits** on the hands or feet.

  c. **Fragile X (Martin-Bell) syndrome**
     – is an X-linked recessively inherited trait characterized by moderate mental retardation.
     – Incidence is approximately 1:1500 male births, and approximately 1:3000 female births.
     – is **second most common genetic cause of moderate mental retardation in males** (trisomy 21 is most common).

4. **Multifactorial (MFD) or polygenic defects**
   – are those defects that involve two or more genes coupled with a strong interaction with environmental factors (e.g., teratogenic drugs or industrial chemicals).
   – are responsible for 25% of major congenital anomalies.
   a. **Neural tube defects (dysraphic states)**
      – are induced by damage occurring in week 4 of fetal development.
      – include spina bifida, encephalocele, myeloschisis with rachischisis, and anencephaly.
      – may be diagnosed prenatally by the presence of **elevated alpha-fetoprotein** levels in the maternal serum and amniotic fluid.
   b. **Cleft lip and cleft palate**
   c. **Cardiovascular anomalies**
   d. **Cryptorchidism** (failure of a testicle to descend)
   e. **Hip dysplasia**

5. **Genetics of Alzheimer disease**
   – One form of Alzheimer disease is an autosomal dominant hereditary disorder.
   – Gene loci have been found on chromosomes 14, 19, and 21.

III. Infectious Agents

  – may be viral or nonviral; bacteria appear to play an insignificant role in congenital anomalies.

  A. **Viral infections**
     – may reach the fetus via the amniotic cavity following vaginal infection, or transplacentally via the bloodstream following maternal viremia.
     1. **Rubella (German measles)**
        – Effects on the developing embryo or fetus may include the triad of **heart defects, cataracts** and **deafness**; in addition, anomalies such as mental retardation, microcephaly, optic atrophy (blindness), and glaucoma may occur.
        – Cardiac defects include patent ductus arteriosus and atrial and ventricular septal defects.
        – Infection during the **embryonic period (weeks 3–8)** results in the **most severe** abnormalities.
     2. **Cytomegalovirus**
        – is the most common of known fetal infections.

- Incidence of women infected during pregnancy is about 3.5%.
- is the cause of **cytomegalic inclusion disease**, which affects primarily the **central nervous system (CNS)**.
- Effects on the developing embryo or fetus may include mental retardation, microcephaly, cerebral calcifications, blindness and chorioretinitis, and hepatosplenomegaly.

3. Herpes simplex virus (HSV)

- The neonate usually acquires HSV in passage through the birth canal of the mother who has **genital herpes**.
- Approximately 50% of newborns delivered vaginally to mothers who have genital herpes contract neonatal herpes; about 50% of newborns with herpes die.
- Infection of the fetus may result in mental retardation, microcephaly, microphthalmia, retinal dysplasia, and hepatosplenomegaly.
- Women with herpes genitalis have a higher risk of developing carcinoma of the vulva and cervix than those not infected.

4. Varicella-zoster virus

- causes **chickenpox** and **shingles**.
- Infection during the first trimester may result in mental retardation, skin scarring, muscle atrophy, limb hypoplasia, and rudimentary digits.

5. Human immunodeficiency virus (HIV)

- may be related to acquired immunodeficiency syndrome (**AIDS**).
- does not appear to cause any major congenital malformations.

B. Nonviral infections

1. Toxoplasma gondii

- is an intracellular **protozoan parasite** that invades the fetus transplacentally.
- is most destructive during the fetal period.
- Congenital defects include mental retardation, hydrocephalus, microcephaly, microphthalmia, chorioretinitis, and intracranial calcifications.
- Pregnant women should avoid cats because they serve as reservoirs of this parasite.

2. Treponema pallidum

- is a **spirochete**, the causative organism of **syphilis**.
- may be transmitted by venereal contact or by the infected mother to the fetus in utero.
- Signs of congenital syphilis develop only in fetuses infected in the latter half of pregnancy.
- The fetus is protected against infection during the first 4 months because of the presence of the Langhans' cell layer of the developing placenta, which is a barrier to transplacental passage of treponemes.
- **Congenital syphilis** may result in mental retardation, hydrocephalus, deafness, corneal opacity and blindness, and abnormal teeth (Hutchinson teeth) and bones.

IV. Drugs, Hormones, and Chemical Agents

A. Prescription drugs

1. Thalidomide

– is an **antinauseant** prescribed for pregnant women (no longer used).
– Congenital defects include malformation of the limbs (meromelia and amelia), heart and kidney defects, intestinal atresia, and atresia of the external acoustic meatus.

2. Antimetabolites (antineoplastic agents)

– are tumor-inhibiting drugs that are highly teratogenic.

a. Aminopterin

– is a folic acid antagonist used to induce therapeutic abortion.
– causes congenital defects such as intrauterine growth retardation, anencephaly, meningocele, hydrocephalus, and cleft lip and cleft palate.

b. Methotrexate

– is a derivative of aminopterin; is also a folic acid antagonist.
– causes multiple **skeletal anomalies**.

3. Diphenylhydantoin (phenytoin [Dilantin])

– is an **anticonvulsant** used to treat epileptic women.
– causes **fetal hydantoin syndrome**, which includes mental retardation, microcephaly, craniofacial defects, and nail and digital hypoplasia.

4. Lithium carbonate

– is the drug of choice for treatment of manic-depressive disorder.
– when given to pregnant women, can cause **congenital anomalies of the heart and great vessels**.

5. Retinoic acid (vitamin A embryopathy)

– is used orally in the treatment of cystic acne and other chronic dermatoses.
– causes craniofacial anomalies, spina bifida cystica, and cardiovascular defects.

6. Warfarin

– is a congener of dicumarol.
– is an oral anticoagulant and a vitamin K antagonist that is used to treat thromboembolic disease.
– **crosses the placental barrier** (heparin does not).
– causes chondrodysplasia, stippled epiphyses, mental retardation, microcephaly, and optic atrophy.

7. Diazepam

– is an antianxiety agent.
– use in the first trimester of pregnancy causes **craniofacial deformities** (cleft lip and cleft palate).

8. Antibiotics

a. Tetracyclines

– cause stained teeth and hypoplasia of enamel and reduced growth of long bones.

b. Streptomycin

– causes sensorineural deafness.

B. Nonprescription drugs and cigarette smoking

1. Alcohol abuse during pregnancy

– is the most common cause of mental retardation.

– results in **fetal alcohol syndrome**.

– results in congenital anomalies such as mental retardation, microcephaly, craniofacial abnormalities (hypertelorism, long philtrum, and short palpebral fissures), limb deformities, and cardiovascular defects (ventricular septal defects); may cause holoprosencephaly.

2. Cigarette smoking

– by pregnant women is a cause of intrauterine growth retardation, premature delivery, and low birth weight.

– The **nicotine** and **carbon monoxide** found in cigarette smoke result in decreased uterine blood flow and diminished capacity of the blood to transport oxygen to the fetal tissue (**fetal hypoxia**).

3. Caffeine

– is not known to be a human teratogen.

4. Potassium iodide

– is found in cough medicine mixtures.

– **crosses the placental membrane**.

– causes thyroid enlargement (goiter) and mental retardation (cretinism).

C. Synthetic steroid hormones

1. Ethisterone and norethisterone

– are synthetic progestins and androgenic agents.

– at one time were prescribed for pregnant women to prevent abortion.

– cause masculinization of the genitalia in female embryos (e.g., enlarged clitoris).

– cause hypospadias in male fetuses.

– use is associated with an increased incidence of cardiovascular anomalies.

2. Diethylstilbestrol (DES)

– is a synthetic estrogen that was used to prevent spontaneous abortion.

– causes congenital abnormalities of the vagina and uterus in women who were exposed to DES in utero; these women are subject to increased risk of contracting adenocarcinoma of the vagina.

3. Oral contraceptives (progestogens and estrogens)

– are teratogenic in pregnant women.

– may cause **VACTERL syndrome**, consisting of: **V**ertebral, **A**nal, **C**ardiac, **T**racheo**E**sophageal, **R**enal, and **L**imb malformations.

D. Illicit drugs

1. Lysergic acid diethylamide (LSD), marijuana, and phencyclidine (PCP, angel dust)

– have not been proven to be teratogenic in humans.

2. Cocaine
- may cause mental retardation, microcephaly, cerebral infarction, and urogenital defects.

E. Chemical agents

1. Organic mercury (methylmercury)
- has been found in contaminated fish and pigs.
- is the cause of Minamata disease.
- **may cross the placental membrane** and cause mental retardation, spasticity, blindness, and seizures.

2. Lead
- **may cross the placental membrane** and cause spontaneous abortion, fetal anomalies, intrauterine growth retardation, and behavioral and psychomotor dysfunction.

3. Polychlorinated biphenyls (PCBs)
- are found in contaminated sport fish.
- are human teratogenic substances that cause intrauterine growth retardation and skin discoloration.

V. Ionizing Radiation

- effect on the embryo or on the fetus depends on the absorbed dose, the dosage, and the stage of development of the embryo or fetus.
- may cause **structural chromosomal damage** (e.g., chromosome breakage).
- may result in congenital anomalies such as mental retardation, microcephaly, spina bifida cystica, cataracts, cleft palate, and skeletal and visceral defects.

VI. Other Factors

A. Mechanical pressure
- Increase in intrauterine pressure may result in congenital anomalies.
- Congenital dislocation of the hip and talipes equinovarus (clubfoot) may result from mechanical pressure, perhaps within a malformed uterus.

B. Prenatal or perinatal hypoxia and asphyxia
- are the most common causes of **cerebral palsy**.

C. Nutrition
- Congenital malformations result after administration of folate antagonists, and also may result from vitamin deficiencies.

D. Parity
- plays a role in the incidence of certain birth defects. For example, **neural tube defects** (spina bifida, anencephaly, and hydrocephalus) and **congenital hip dislocation** occur with greater frequency in firstborn infants.

E. Age of the pregnant mother
- See II A 1 a.

F. Maternal hyperthermia

– is caused by viral pyrogenic infection, and may cause **neural tube defects** (anencephaly).

– Hot-tub bathing may cause congenital anomalies of the CNS.

G. Maternal diabetes

– Incidence of congenital anomalies in the children of diabetic mothers is much higher than in children of nondiabetic mothers.

– may cause congenital anomalies such as cardiac and skeletal defects and neural tube defects.

– is associated with the **caudal regression syndrome**: dysgenesis or agenesis of the sacral vertebrae and hindlimb hypoplasia.

H. Failure of neural crest cells to migrate

1. DiGeorge syndrome

– is a nongenetic form of T-cell deficiency.

– results from failure of the neural crest cells to populate pharyngeal pouches 3 and 4 and give rise to the thymus and parathyroid glands.

– is characterized by congenital hypothyroidism and facial and cardiac abnormalities.

2. Cardiac malformations

– result from failure of neural crest cells to migrate to the heart and form the aorticopulmonary (AP) septum.

3. Hirschsprung disease (congenital aganglionic megacolon) [see Chapters 7 and 10]

Review Test

Directions: Each of the numbered items or incomplete statements in this section is followed by answers or by completions of the statement. Select the **one** lettered answer or completion that is **best** in each case.

1. What percentage of liveborn infants have defects at birth?

(A) 1%
(B) 3%
(C) 5%
(D) 10%
(E) 15%

2. What percent of infant deaths in the United States result from congenital malformations?

(A) 5%
(B) 10%
(C) 15%
(D) 20%
(E) 30%

3. The most common viral infection in the human fetus is caused by the

(A) cytomegalovirus (CMV)
(B) herpes simplex virus (HSV)
(C) human immunodeficiency virus (HIV)
(D) rubella virus
(E) varicella-zoster virus

4. The incidence of trisomy 21 in babies born to women over the age of 45 is

(A) 1:25
(B) 1:100
(C) 1:800
(D) 1:1000
(E) 1:10000

5. The second most common inherited cause of moderate mental retardation in males is caused by

(A) trisomy 18
(B) trisomy 13
(C) Turner syndrome
(D) triple X syndrome
(E) fragile X syndrome

6. A tall, male eunuchoid patient with hyalinization of the seminiferous tubules, testicular atrophy, and gynecomastia would best match with which one of the following chromosome complements?

(A) 47,XXY
(B) 47,XYY
(C) 48,XXXX
(D) 48,XXYY
(E) 49,XXXYY

7. All of the following environmental agents may cause microcephaly and mental retardation EXCEPT

(A) aminopterin
(B) diphenylhydantoin
(C) thalidomide
(D) warfarin
(E) x-rays

8. Which of the following congenital anomalies is a single-gene defect?

(A) Achondroplasia
(B) Anencephaly
(C) Cleft palate
(D) Hip dysplasia
(E) Spina bifida

9. Elevated alpha-fetoprotein levels in the amniotic fluid or in the maternal serum is found in which one of the following malformations?

(A) Achondroplasia
(B) Anencephaly
(C) Cryptorchidism
(D) Esophagotracheal fistula
(E) Tetralogy of Fallot

Directions: Each group of items in this section consists of lettered options followed by a set of numbered items. For each item, select the **one** lettered option that is most closely associated with it. Each lettered option may be selected once, more than once, or not at all.

Questions 10–14

Match the characteristic with the infectious agent associated with it.

(A) Rubella
(B) Cytomegalovirus
(C) Herpes simplex virus
(D) *Toxoplasma gondii*
(E) *Treponema pallidum*

10. Fetal protection against this infection during the first 4 months is because of the presence of the Langhans' cell layer of developing placenta

11. Is associated with the triad of heart defects, cataracts, and deafness

12. Is the most common cause of fetal infection

13. Cats are frequent reservoirs of this organism

14. Produces its most severe damage during the embryonic period

Questions 15–19

Match the characteristic with the syndrome associated with it.

(A) Cri du chat syndrome
(B) Down syndrome
(C) Edwards' syndrome
(D) Patau syndrome
(E) Turner syndrome

15. Results from a sex chromosome abnormality

16. Characterized by prominent occiput, low-set ears, micrognathia, flexed digits, and rocker-bottom feet

17. Is the classic form of gonadal dysgenesis

18. Results from deletion of the short arm of chromosome 5

19. Is associated with the pathology of Alzheimer disease

Answers and Explanations

1–B. Approximately 3% of liveborn infants have defects at birth. This statistic doubles by the end of the first year of life.

2–D. Approximately 20% of deaths that occur during the neonatal period result from congenital malformations.

3–A. CMV causes cytomegalic inclusion disease. It is the most common of known fetal infections. CMV infection in the first trimester usually results in spontaneous abortion; in the late fetal period, CMV infection may result in mental retardation, blindness, deafness, and cerebral palsy. Rubella infections have decreased since the development of an attenuated rubella virus vaccine.

4–A. The incidence of Down syndrome in babies born to women over the age of 45 is 1:25. The incidence in the general population is 1:800.

5–E. The second most common inherited cause of moderate mental retardation in males is caused by fragile X syndrome, or Martin-Bell syndrome (Down syndrome is the most common). Fragile X syndrome occurs in approximately 1:2000 male births and in approximately 1:3000 female births.

6–A. The tall, male eunuchoid patient with hyalinization of the seminiferous tubules, testicular atrophy, and gynecomastia has Klinefelter syndrome. His somatic cells have 47 chromosomes and a sex chromosomal complement of the XXY type. This syndrome represents a trisomy of sex chromosomes. In most cases, a Barr (sex chromatin) body is found. The approximate incidence is 1:1000 in male births. These patients often have educational problems. They are all sterile.

7–C. Aminopterin, diphenylhydantoin (Dilantin), warfarin, and x-rays are all teratogens that produce congenital anomalies; they all are known to produce microcephaly. Thalidomide is a dangerous teratogen that produces limb defects (amelia and meromelia) and cardiac abnormalities; it does not cause microcephaly. Use of thalidomide in pregnant women has been discontinued.

8–A. Achondroplasia, polydactyly, and the fragile X syndrome are single-gene defects. Anencephaly, spina bifida, cleft palate, and hip dysplasia are caused by multifactorial inheritance.

9–B. Elevated alpha-fetoprotein levels in the amniotic fluid or in the maternal serum are found in anencephaly, a neural tube defect. Neural tube defects also include spina bifida.

10–E. The fetus is protected against infection by *Treponema pallidum* during the first 4 months of gestation because of the presence of the Langhans' cell layer of the developing placenta, which is a barrier to transplacental passage of treponemas.

11–A. Rubella is associated with the triad of heart defects, cataracts, and deafness (congenital rubella syndrome). In addition, rubella also causes mental retardation, optic atrophy (blindness), and glaucoma. The heart defects include patent ductus arteriosus and atrial and ventricular septal defects.

12–B. The cytomegalovirus is the most common cause of fetal infections; incidence of women infected during pregnancy is about 3.5%.

13–D. Cats are frequent reservoirs for the protozoan *Toxoplasma gondii*. Women should avoid touching cats during pregnancy.

14–A. Rubella produces its severest effects when active during the embryonic period.

15–E. Turner syndrome (45,Xo) is a sex chromosome abnormality occurring only in females. It is also called monosomy X chromosome syndrome. It is also the classic form of gonadal dysgenesis.

16–C. Edwards' syndrome (trisomy 18) is characterized by prominent occiput, low-set ears, micrognathia, flexed digits, and rocker-bottom feet. In addition mental retardation and congenital heart defects are seen.

17–E. Turner syndrome is the classic form of gonadal dysgenesis; patients are mentally retarded and have infantile genitalia, hypoplastic ovaries, congenital heart defects, webbed neck, and lymphedema of the extremities. Various mosaics can occur.

18–A. Cri du chat syndrome is classified as a structural chromosomal abnormality, which results from deletion of the short arm of chromosome 5. It is characterized by mental retardation, microcephaly, congenital heart defects, and a cat-like cry.

19–B. Trisomy 21 (Down syndrome) is the most common type of trisomy. Persons with Down syndrome over 30 years of age demonstrate the same neuropathology as Alzheimer patients: neurofibrillary tangles and neuritic plaques.

Comprehensive Examination

Directions: Each of the numbered items or incomplete statements in this section is followed by answers or by completions of the statement. Select the **one** lettered answer or completion that is **best** in each case.

1. The second meiotic division is characterized by which of the following events?

(A) Crossing over
(B) Cell division
(C) Alignment
(D) Centromere splitting
(E) Synapsis

2. One primary oocyte will give rise to which of the following cells?

(A) 1 mature ovum and 3 polar bodies
(B) 1 immature oogonium
(C) 4 mature ova
(D) 16 mature ova
(E) 32 mature ova

3. A 40-year-old woman becomes pregnant. For approximately how long was the primary oocyte that formed the ovum arrested in prophase of meiosis I?

(A) 48 hours
(B) 1 week
(C) 1 month
(D) 12 years
(E) 40 years

4. At the beginning of week 2 of human development, which of the following germ layers is present?

(A) Epiblast
(B) Hypoblast
(C) Epiblast and hypoblast
(D) Epiblast and mesoderm
(E) Ectoderm and mesoderm

5. Human chorionic gonadotropin (hCG) can first be assayed in the maternal urine

(A) at day 8 after fertilization
(B) at day 10 after fertilization
(C) at day 14 after fertilization
(D) during the early fetal period
(E) during the late fetal period

6. A young woman was exposed to the rubella virus during pregnancy, which resulted in her baby having a ventriculoseptal cardiac defect. In which period was the mother most likely to have contracted the acute viral infection?

(A) Weeks 1–5 before fertilization
(B) Weeks 1–5 after fertilization
(C) Months 4–5 after fertilization
(D) Months 5–6 after fertilization
(E) Months 6–7 after fertilization

7. In the human embryo, hematopoiesis first occurs during week 3 of development within the

(A) liver
(B) bone marrow
(C) spleen
(D) yolk sac
(E) primitive heart tube

8. The process of gastrulation is first indicated by the formation of the

(A) prochordal plate
(B) cloacal membrane
(C) primitive streak
(D) neural tube
(E) somites

9. The notochord induces the overlying ectoderm to develop into the

(A) skin
(B) eye
(C) primitive streak
(D) primitive node
(E) neural plate

10. A sacrococcygeal teratoma is a tumor that arises from remnants of the

(A) neural plate
(B) cloacal membrane
(C) posterior neuropore
(D) primitive streak
(E) notochord

11. Unequal division of the truncus arteriosus by the aorticopulmonary (AP) septum will most likely result in

(A) patent ductus arteriosus
(B) patent foramen ovale
(C) coarctation of the aorta
(D) pulmonary stenosis
(E) interventricular septal defect

12. During a surgical procedure for ligation of a patent ductus arteriosus, which nerve is likely to be damaged?

(A) Hypoglossal nerve (CN XII)
(B) Glossopharyngeal nerve (CN IX)
(C) Phrenic nerve
(D) Left recurrent laryngeal nerve
(E) Right recurrent laryngeal nerve

13. Coarctation of the aorta proximal to the ligamentum arteriosum is likely to involve which aortic arch?

(A) Aortic arch 2
(B) Aortic arch 3
(C) Aortic arch 4
(D) Aortic arch 5
(E) Aortic arch 6

14. The ductus arteriosus is derived from which one of the following aortic arches?

(A) Right aortic arch 4
(B) Left aortic arch 4
(C) Right aortic arch 5
(D) Right aortic arch 6
(E) Left aortic arch 6

15. Which of the following structures is the fetal component of the placenta?

(A) Decidua capsularis
(B) Decidua parietalis
(C) Decidua basalis
(D) Secondary chorionic villi
(E) Tertiary chorionic villi

16. The placenta can be considered an endocrine gland because it secretes which of the following hormones?

(A) Human chorionic gonadotropin (hCG)
(B) Human placental lactogen (hPL)
(C) Progesterone
(D) Estrogen
(E) All of the above

17. The anterior lobe of the pituitary gland is derived from

(A) the epithalamus
(B) the hypothalamus
(C) the ventral thalamus
(D) Rathke's pouch
(E) the proctodeum

18. Which of the following tumors is associated with Rathke's pouch?

(A) Cholesteatoma
(B) Chordoma
(C) Craniopharyngioma
(D) Medulloblastoma
(E) Pituitary adenoma

19. The neurohypophysis is derived from the

(A) epithalamus
(B) hypothalamus
(C) metathalamus
(D) stomodeum
(E) subthalamus

20. Agenesis of the lamina terminalis results in which one of the following congenital defects?

(A) Anencephaly
(B) Arhinencephaly
(C) Diastematomyelia
(D) Hydranencephaly
(E) Spina bifida

21. The space of retinal detachment (the intraretinal space) lies between the

(A) outer nuclear layer and the inner nuclear layer
(B) inner nuclear layer and the ganglion cell layer
(C) layer of rods and cones and the pigment epithelial layer
(D) ganglion cell layer and the layer of optic nerve fibers
(E) pigment epithelial layer and the choriocapillaris layer of the choroid

22. Which of the following adult structures is derived from the ventral mesentery?

(A) Greater omentum
(B) Falciform ligament
(C) Ligamentum venosum
(D) Ligamentum arteriosum
(E) Median umbilical ligament

23. Which of the following adult structures is a remnant of the left umbilical vein?

(A) Falciform ligament
(B) Ligamentum venosum
(C) Ligamentum arteriosum
(D) Median umbilical ligament
(E) Ligamentum teres hepatis

24. Surfactant begins to form in the human fetus at

(A) week 2
(B) week 5
(C) week 13
(D) week 24
(E) birth

25. An obstruction of the pharynx in a neonate caused by a large mass located on the posterior part of the tongue near the foramen cecum is most likely caused by

(A) ectopic lymphoid tissue
(B) ectopic thymic tissue
(C) ectopic thyroid tissue
(D) ectopic parathyroid tissue
(E) swollen tonsils

26. Treacher Collins syndrome occurs when which of the following pharyngeal arches develops abnormally?

(A) Pharyngeal arch 1
(B) Pharyngeal arch 2
(C) Pharyngeal arch 3
(D) Pharyngeal arch 4
(E) Pharyngeal arch 6

27. Which of the following structures is involved in the formation of a cleft palate?

(A) Pharyngeal arch 2
(B) Pharyngeal arch 3
(C) The palatine shelves
(D) The frontonasal prominence
(E) The maxillary prominence and medial nasal prominence

28. Which of the following structures is involved in the formation of a cleft lip?

(A) Pharyngeal arch 2
(B) Pharyngeal arch 3
(C) The palatine shelves
(D) The frontonasal prominence
(E) The maxillary prominence and medial nasal prominence

29. The prostate gland is derived from

(A) the allantois
(B) the paramesonephric duct
(C) the mesonephric duct
(D) endodermal outgrowths from the urethra
(E) endodermal outgrowths from the yolk sac

30. A pheochromocytoma is a tumor consisting of chromaffin cells, which secrete epinephrine, and is generally associated with the adrenal medulla. Embryologically, chromaffin cells are derived from

(A) ectoderm
(B) mesoderm
(C) endoderm
(D) visceral mesoderm
(E) neural crest cells

31. The adult ureter is derived from the stalk of the ureteric bud. The ureteric bud develops as an outgrowth of the

(A) metanephric blastema
(B) mesonephric duct
(C) metanephric vesicle
(D) pronephric duct
(E) mesonephric tubules

32. The transitional epithelium lining the adult urinary bladder is derived from which one of the following structures?

(A) Midgut
(B) Foregut
(C) Mesonephric duct
(D) Paramesonephric duct
(E) Urogenital sinus

33. Incomplete fusion of the urethral folds in the male results in a condition known as

(A) epispadias
(B) hypospadias
(C) cryptorchidism
(D) hydrocele
(E) bifid penis

34. Failure of the testes to descend into the scrotum within 3 months after birth results in a condition known as

(A) epispadias
(B) hypospadias
(C) cryptorchidism
(D) hydrocele
(E) bifid penis

35. Which of the following statements concerning the development of the reproductive system in the female is correct?

(A) The clitoris is analogous to the penis
(B) The urethral folds fail to fuse
(C) The urethral folds form the labia minora
(D) The labia majora is analogous to the scrotum
(E) All of the above

36. The positional changes of the diaphragm in the developing embryo are most clearly demonstrated by

(A) its vascular supply
(B) its innervation by the phrenic nerve
(C) its lymphatic supply
(D) its 270° counterclockwise rotation
(E) its relationship to the common cardinal veins

37. Fetal sex determination using ultrasonography is first possible in which week after fertilization?

(A) Week 8
(B) Week 12
(C) Week 14
(D) Week 16
(E) Week 18

38. Which one of the following substances has been shown to be a teratogen?

(A) Caffeine
(B) Cocaine
(C) Lysergic acid diethylamide (LSD)
(D) Marijuana
(E) Phencyclidine (angel dust)

Questions 39–42

A premature infant weighing 1250 grams develops rapid, shallow respirations with an associated grunting noise and becomes cyanotic. Chest x-rays show dense lungs and atelectasis.

39. What is the most likely diagnosis?

(A) Tetralogy of Fallot
(B) Tracheoesophageal fistula
(C) Congenital diaphragmatic hernia
(D) Respiratory distress syndrome
(E) Bronchiectasis

40. The best predictive prenatal laboratory test for this condition is

(A) karyotype analysis
(B) measurement of amniotic fluid volume
(C) measurement of lecithin/sphingomyelin (L/S) ratio
(D) genetic screening of the entire family
(E) measurement of alpha-fetoprotein level

41. Which cell type is most specifically involved in this condition?

(A) Type I pneumocyte
(B) Type II pneumocyte
(C) Podocyte
(D) Goblet cell
(E) Paneth cell

42. If this condition is diagnosed during the pregnancy, the most beneficial drug treatment to administer to the mother would be

(A) diazepam
(B) vitamin B
(C) antibiotics
(D) insulin
(E) steroids

43. All of the following structures are components of a human blastocyst capable of implantation EXCEPT

(A) the blastocyst cavity
(B) the embryoblast
(C) the cytotrophoblast
(D) the syncytiotrophoblast
(E) the zona pellucida

44. All of the following statements concerning fetal circulation are true EXCEPT

(A) the left umbilical vein carries highly oxygenated blood to the fetus
(B) the umbilical arteries carry poorly oxygenated blood to the placenta
(C) only a minimal amount of blood goes to the lungs
(D) the ductus venosus carries poorly oxygenated blood
(E) blood from the right atrium passes to the left atrium via the foramen ovale

45. All of the following substances are readily transferred across the placental membrane EXCEPT

(A) water
(B) rubella virus
(C) succinylcholine
(D) cocaine
(E) alcohol

46. All of the following structures are derived from the rhombic lips EXCEPT

(A) the dentate nucleus
(B) the emboliform nucleus
(C) the fastigial nucleus
(D) the globose nucleus
(E) the gracile nucleus

47. The surface ectoderm gives rise to all of the following structures EXCEPT

(A) the lens placode
(B) the otic placode
(C) the utricle
(D) the spiral organ of Corti
(E) the dilator pupillae muscle

48. A newborn infant with DiGeorge syndrome will display all of the following characteristics EXCEPT

(A) lack of thymic tissue
(B) lack of parathyroid tissue
(C) cleft lip
(D) facial anomalies
(E) cardiovascular anomalies

49. All of the following are characteristics of testicular feminization syndrome EXCEPT

(A) 46,XY genotype
(B) presence of female external genitalia
(C) lack of uterus and uterine tubes
(D) presence of testes
(E) presence of ovaries

50. The definitive adult diaphragm is formed embryologically from all of the following structures EXCEPT

(A) pleuropericardial membranes
(B) septum transversum
(C) pleuroperitoneal membranes
(D) dorsal mesentery of the esophagus
(E) body wall

Directions: Each group of items in this section consists of lettered options followed by a set of numbered items. For each item, select the **one** lettered option that is most closely associated with it. Each lettered option may be selected once, more than once, or not at all.

Questions 51–58

Match each descriptive phrase with the appropriate cardiac anomaly.

(A) Tetralogy of Fallot
(B) Membranous ventricular septal defect (VSD)
(C) Persistent truncus arteriosus
(D) Transposition of the great arteries
(E) Foramen secundum defect
(F) Coarctation of the aorta
(G) Patent ductus arteriosus
(H) Tricuspid atresia

51. Results in a large opening between the right and left atria

52. Is characterized by a patent foramen ovale, interventricular (IV) septal defect, overdeveloped left ventricle, and underdeveloped right ventricle

53. Aorta originates from the right ventricle; the pulmonary trunk originates from the left ventricle

54. Is characterized by pulmonary stenosis, overriding aorta, interventricular (IV) septal defect, and right ventricular hypertrophy

55. Is the most common congenital cardiac malformation

56. A single arterial vessel leaves the heart and gives rise to the pulmonary trunk and aorta

57. Lumen of the aorta is constricted below the origin of the left subclavian artery

58. Functionally closes within a few hours after birth

Questions 59–70

Match each description with the appropriate nerve.

(A) Olfactory nerve (CN I)
(B) Optic nerve (CN II)
(C) Oculomotor nerve (CN III)
(D) Trochlear nerve (CN IV)
(E) Trigeminal nerve (CN V)
(F) Abducent nerve (CN VI)
(G) Facial nerve (CN VII)
(H) Vestibulocochlear nerve (CN VIII)
(I) Glossopharyngeal nerve (CN IX)
(J) Vagus nerve (CN X)
(K) Accessory nerve (CN XI)
(L) Hypoglossal nerve (CN XII)

59. Innervates the structures of pharyngeal arches 4 and 6

60. Is derived from the basal plate of the rostral midbrain

61. Innervates the structures of pharyngeal arch 1

62. Is derived from the diencephalon

63. Innervates the structures of pharyngeal arch 3

64. Arises from the only general somatic efferent (GSE) nucleus of the medulla

65. Is derived from the basal plate of the caudal midbrain

66. Innervates the structures of pharyngeal arch 2

67. Arises from the only general somatic efferent (GSE) nucleus of the pons

68. Is derived from the otic placode

69. Innervates the muscles of the occipital somites

70. Innervates muscles derived from the preotic myotomes and a muscle derived from the neuroectoderm

Questions 71–76

Match each description with the appropriate condition.

(A) Anencephaly
(B) Arnold-Chiari syndrome
(C) Dandy-Walker syndrome
(D) Holoprosencephaly
(E) Hydranencephaly

71. A huge intracerebral cavitation resulting from infarction in the territory of the internal carotid artery

72. Commonly seen in trisomy 13 (Patau syndrome)

73. Fusion of frontal lobes and agenesis of olfactory bulbs

74. Failure of anterior neuropore to close

75. Atresia of the outlet foramina of the fourth ventricle

76. Herniation of caudal vermis and cerebellar tonsils through the foramen magnum

Questions 77–81

Match each description with the appropriate membrane.

(A) Vestibular membrane
(B) Iridopupillary membrane
(C) Tympanic membrane
(D) Tectorial membrane
(E) Basilar membrane

77. Separates the cochlear duct from the scala tympani

78. Found in an endolymphatic space

79. Usually not found after birth

80. Is in contact with hair cells

81. Derived from three germ layers

Questions 82–86

Match each description of an otic structure with the appropriate lettered structure in the illustration.

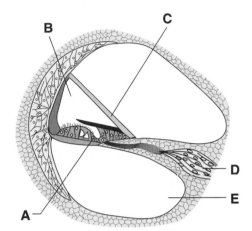

Modified from Johnson KE: *Human Developmental Anatomy.* Baltimore, Williams & Wilkins, 1988, p 356.

82. Lies within the modiolus

83. Has pitch localization along its length

84. Contains a fluid that communicates with the subarachnoid space

85. Separates the scala vestibuli from the cochlear duct

86. Contains a fluid elaborated by the stria vascularis

Questions 87–91

Match each description of an optic structure with the appropriate lettered structure in the illustration.

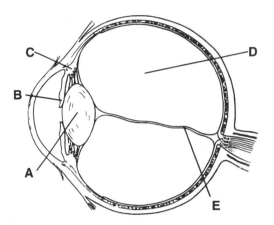

87. Is derived from the neuroectoderm of the optic cup

88. Involved in the production of aqueous humor

89. Is formed by mesodermal cells that migrate through the choroid (optic) fissure, forming a refractive medium

90. A nonfunctional structure in the adult

91. Is derived from the surface ectoderm

Questions 92–97

Match each descriptive statement with the appropriate lettered structure in the illustration.

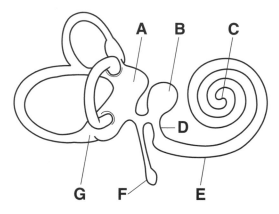

Modified from Johnson KE: *Human Developmental Anatomy.* Baltimore, Williams & Wilkins, 1988, p 348.

92. Contains the macula utriculi

93. Localization of high-pitched sounds

94. Responds to linear acceleration and is connected to the scala media

95. Thought to be the site of endolymph absorption

96. Sensory receptors that respond to angular acceleration

97. Contains the macula sacculi

Directions: Each group of items in this section consists of lettered options followed by a set of numbered items. For each item, select the **one** lettered option that is most closely associated with it. Each lettered option may be selected once, more than once, or not at all.

Questions 98–108

Match each descriptive statement with the appropriate congenital anomaly of the digestive system.

(A) Esophageal atresia
(B) Hypertrophic pyloric stenosis
(C) Extrahepatic biliary atresia
(D) Accelerated development of pancreatic islets
(E) Omphalocele
(F) Ileal (Meckel's) diverticulum
(G) Gastroschisis
(H) Malrotation of the midgut
(I) Hirschsprung's disease
(J) Anal agenesis
(K) Anorectal agenesis

98. Absence of parasympathetic ganglion cells in the myenteric plexus

99. May be associated with a tracheoesophageal fistula

100. Intestines fail to return to the abdominal cavity

101. Generally associated clinically with volvulus

102. Associated with increased birth weight

103. Occurs when a remnant of the vitelline duct persists

104. Associated with projectile vomiting after feeding

105. A defect of the ventral abdominal wall

106. Lumen of the ducts is obliterated due to incomplete recanalization

107. Anal canal ends as a blind sac below the puborectalis muscle

108. Most common type of anorectal malformation

Questions 109–113

Match each structure below with the appropriate pharyngeal arch.

(A) Pharyngeal arch 1
(B) Pharyngeal arch 2
(C) Pharyngeal arch 3
(D) Pharyngeal arch 4
(E) Pharyngeal arch 6

109. Recurrent laryngeal nerve

110. Superior laryngeal nerve

111. Muscles of facial expression

112. Muscles of mastication

113. Constrictor muscles of the pharynx

Questions 114–118

Match each description with the appropriate skull abnormality.

(A) Acromegaly
(B) Microcephaly
(C) Oxycephaly
(D) Plagiocephaly
(E) Scaphocephaly

114. Mental retardation

115. May follow exposure to infections in utero

116. Large jaw, hands, and feet

117. A long skull

118. A towerlike skull

Questions 119–123

Match each description below with the appropriate lettered structure in the illustration.

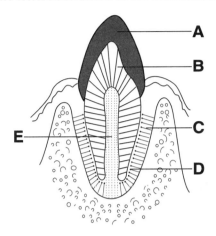

119. Formed by cementoblasts

120. Formed by cells derived from the neural crest

121. Formed by ameloblasts

122. Formed by odontoblasts

123. Formed by cells derived from ectoderm

Questions 124–131

Match each description below with the appropriate substance.

(A) Alpha-fetoprotein
(B) Aminopterin
(C) Human chorionic gonadotropin (hCG)
(D) Diazepam
(E) Potassium iodide
(F) Retinoic acid
(G) Streptomycin
(H) Unconjugated estriol

124. An anxiolytic agent that may cause cleft lip and cleft palate

125. May cause sensorineural deafness

126. An oral antiacne medication that may cause neural tube defects and cardiovascular anomalies

127. Maternal serum level of this hormone reduced when fetus has Down syndrome

128. Low maternal serum level of this non-hormone associated with trisomy 21

129. High maternal serum values associated with neural tube defects

130. Intrauterine growth retardation, anencephaly, spina bifida, hydrocephalus, and cleft lip and palate

131. Thyroid hyperplasia and mental retardation (cretinism)

Questions 132–136

Match each description with the appropriate syndrome.

(A) Angelman syndrome
(B) DiGeorge syndrome
(C) Down syndrome
(D) Prader-Willi syndrome
(E) VACTERL syndrome

132. Characterized by neuritic plaques and neurofibrillary tangles

133. Associated with the use of oral contraceptives during pregnancy

134. Characterized by an absence of the thymus and parathyroid glands and T-cell insufficiency

135. Associated with a chromosome deletion in the father

136. Associated with a chromosome deletion in the mother

Answers and Explanations

1–D. The second meiotic division (meiosis II) is characterized by centromere splitting. Meiosis is a specialized process of cell division that occurs only in the production of gametes. The process consists of two divisions (meiosis I and meiosis II) that result in the formation of four gametes, each containing half the number of chromosomes (23 chromosomes) and half the amount of DNA (1N) found in normal somatic cells.

2–A. A primary oocyte will give rise to one mature ovum and three nonfunctional polar bodies.

3–E. The primary oocyte that matured to become the fertilized ovum in this woman remained dormant in prophase of meiosis I for 40 years. Proliferation of oogonia and their differentiation to primary oocytes are completed before birth. All primary oocytes are formed by the fifth month of fetal life and remain arrested in prophase of meiosis I at least until puberty; then from 5 to 15 primary oocytes will begin maturation with each ovarian cycle.

4–C. At week 2 of development, the epiblast and hypoblast form a flat, ovoid-shaped disk known as the bilaminar embryonic disk.

5–B. Human chorionic gonadotropin (hCG), which is produced by the syncytiotrophoblast, can be assayed in the maternal urine at day 10 after fertilization and in maternal blood at day 8. Over-the-counter early pregnancy testing kits diagnose pregnancy based on the presence of this hormone.

6–B. Anomalies related to the congenital rubella syndrome—including cardiac defects, cataracts, and deafness—are seen most commonly in infants who were exposed to the viral infection during weeks 1–5 after fertilization. During this period the heart, brain, eye, and ear of the embryo are highly sensitive to various teratogens. The risk of congenital anomalies due to rubella infection during the second and third trimesters is low.

7–D. Blood cell formation (hematopoiesis) first occurs within the extraembryonic visceral mesoderm surrounding the yolk sac. Beginning at week 5, hematopoiesis is taken over by a sequence of embryonic organs: liver, spleen, thymus, and bone marrow.

8–C. The process of gastrulation is first indicated by the formation of the primitive streak.

9–E. The notochord induces the overlying ectoderm to differentiate into the neural plate.

10–D. The primitive streak normally degenerates and disappears. If remnants persist, the pluripotential cells of the primitive streak can form a sacrococcygeal teratoma.

11–D. Abnormal neural crest cell migration may result in the formation of a skewed aorticopulmonary (AP) septum. This usually causes pulmonary stenosis; it sometimes causes pulmonary atresia if the AP septum is skewed badly.

12–D. The left recurrent laryngeal nerve may be damaged during ligation of a patent ductus arteriosus. Early in development, both the right and left recurrent laryngeal nerves hook around aortic arch 6. On the right side, the distal part of aortic arch 6 regresses, and the right recurrent laryngeal nerve moves up to hook around the right subclavian artery. On the left side, aortic arch 6 persists as the ductus arteriosus; the left recurrent laryngeal nerve remains hooked around the ductus arteriosus.

13–C. The portion of the aorta just proximal to the ligamentum arteriosum is formed from aortic arch 4.

14–E. The ductus arteriosus is derived from left aortic arch 6.

15–E. The fetal component of the placenta consists of the tertiary chorionic villi (or villous chorion). The decidua basalis is the maternal component of the placenta.

16–E. The placenta secretes many hormones, including hCG, hPL, progesterone, estrogen, chorionic thyrotropin (hCT), chorionic adrenocorticotropin (hACTH), prolactin, relaxin, and prostaglandins.

17–D. The anterior lobe of the pituitary gland is derived from Rathke's pouch, an ectodermal diverticulum of the primitive mouth cavity (the stomodeum). The posterior lobe of the pituitary gland is derived from the infundibulum, a diverticulum of the hypothalamus.

18–C. Craniopharyngiomas, tumors associated with Rathke's pouch, represent the most common supratentorial tumors occurring in childhood. These tumors compress the optic chiasm, the pituitary gland, and the hypothalamus.

19–B. The neurohypophysis, the posterior lobe of the pituitary gland, is derived from an outpocketing of the floor of the hypothalamus. The adenohypophysis, the anterior lobe of the pituitary gland, develops from an outpouching of the stomodeum, the oral cavity. The metathalamus consists of the lateral and medial geniculate bodies.

20–A. Agenesis of the lamina terminalis results in anencephaly; closure of the anterior neuropore results in formation of the lamina terminalis. Diastematomyelia is a sagittal division of the spinal cord.

21–C. Retinal detachment takes place in the space between the layer of rods and cones and the pigment epithelial layer of the choroid.

22–B. The falciform ligament and lesser omentum in the adult are derivatives of the ventral mesentery. The greater omentum forms from the dorsal mesentery. The ligamentum venosum is a remnant of the ductus venosus, which regresses after birth. The ligamentum arteriosum is a remnant of the ductus arteriosus, which connects the pulmonary artery and aorta. The median umbilical ligament is a remnant of the allantois, which becomes a thick fibrous cord in the fetus called the urachus and extends from the apex of the urinary bladder to the umbilicus. In the adult, the urachus is called the median umbilical ligament.

23–E. The left umbilical vein connects with the ductus venosus to return oxygenated blood from the placenta to the developing fetus. After birth, the left umbilical vein regresses and its remnant is known as the ligamentum teres hepatis, or round ligament of the liver.

24–D. Surfactant begins to form during the terminal sac period of lung development, which is between week 24 and birth.

25–C. The thyroid gland forms as an endodermal diverticulum of the foregut. The thyroid diverticulum migrates caudally but remains connected to the tongue by the thyroglossal duct, which opens on the tongue at the foramen cecum.

26–A. Treacher Collins syndrome manifests as severe facial anomalies caused by the lack of neural crest migration into pharyngeal arch 1.

27–C. Failure of the palatine shelves to fuse with the primary palate results in an anterior cleft palate. Failure of the palatine shelves to fuse with each other and with the nasal septum results in a posterior cleft palate.

28–E. Cleft lip occurs when the maxillary prominence and medial nasal prominence fail to fuse and the underlying somitomeric mesoderm and neural crest fail to expand, resulting in a persistent labial groove.

29–D. The prostate gland forms from endodermal outgrowths of the prostatic urethra into the surrounding mesoderm. Initially, about five groups of solid prostatic cords form; by week 11, they develop lumina and glandular acini. The mesoderm differentiates into the smooth muscle and connective tissue of the prostate.

30–E. Chromaffin cells of the adrenal medulla are derived from nearby sympathetic ganglia, which in turn are derived from neural crest cells. At birth, chromaffin cells are found in widely dispersed sites, which undergo involution until puberty. Remnants of these chromaffin cells account for extra-adrenal sites of pheochromocytomas. Clinically, pheochromocytomas are associated with headache, excessive perspiration, palpitations, and hypertension, probably due to the increased levels of epinephrine.

31–B. The ureteric bud develops as an outgrowth of the mesonephric duct. The ureteric bud penetrates the metanephric blastema and undergoes repeated divisions to form the ureter, pelvis, major calyx, minor calyx, and collecting tubules.

32-E. The transitional epithelium lining the urinary bladder is derived from endoderm lining the upper part of the urogenital sinus.

33–B. Fusion of the urethral folds is responsible for the formation of the penile urethra in the male. If incomplete fusion occurs, abnormal openings on the ventral surface of the penis– hypospadias–will be found.

34–C. Cryptorchidism results if the testes fail to descend into the scrotum within 3 months after birth. The undescended testes are generally found in the abdominal cavity or inguinal canal. Bilateral cryptorchidism results in sterility.

35–E. The external genitalia of the female and male form from the same three structures: phallus, urethral folds, and genital swellings. These three structures will be remodeled into the definitive adult external genitalia depending on whether a female or male phenotype is specified genetically.

36–B. During week 4 of development, the diaphragm is innervated by the phrenic nerves, which originate from C3, C4, and C5. By week 8, there is an apparent descent of the diaphragm to L1 due to the rapid growth of the neural tube, and the phrenic nerves are carried along.

37–B. Fetal sex determination using ultrasonography is first possible in week 12 after fertilization, or in week 14 after the last menstrual period. The sex of an aborted fetus cannot be determined by visual examination before week 12.

38–B. Cocaine has been shown to be a teratogenic agent; its use has resulted in mental retardation, microcephaly, cerebral infarction, and urogenital defects.

39–D. A premature infant who presents with shallow, grunting respirations, cyanosis, and dense lungs on chest x-ray has respiratory distress syndrome, which is caused by a deficiency or absence of surfactant.

40–C. The lecithin/sphingomyelin (L/S) ratio has long been the gold standard in fetal lung maturity testing. Surfactant is a surface-active detergent composed of phosphatidylcholine (mainly dipalmitoyl lecithin). Surfactant production begins by week 24 of development, but the substance is present in only small amounts in premature infants. Sphingomyelin levels in amniotic fluid are constant throughout gestation, but the lecithin levels begin to rise at week 28. Other fetal lung maturity tests are available that measure phosphatidylcholine levels specifically.

41–B. The type II pneumocyte is responsible for the production of surfactant.

42–E. Both thyroxine and cortisol stimulate the differentiation of type II pneumocytes and thus increase surfactant levels.

43–E. After the zona pellucida degenerates, the trophoblast differentiates into the cytotrophoblast and syncytiotrophoblast in preparation for implantation.

44–D. Highly oxygenated and nutrient-enriched blood returns to the fetus from the placenta via the left umbilical vein. Some of this blood percolates through the liver, but most bypasses the sinusoids by passing through the ductus venosus and entering the inferior vena cava.

45–C. Muscle relaxants (such as succinylcholine), curare, heparin, and other drugs similar to amino acids (such as methyldopa) do not cross the placental membrane.

46–E. The rhombic lips develop from the alar plates of the rhombencephalon and give rise to the cerebellum and the cerebellar nuclei. The gracile nucleus is derived from the alar plate of the myelencephalon.

47–E. The dilator and sphincter pupillae muscles are derived from the neuroectoderm of the optic cup.

48–C. DiGeorge syndrome is not associated with cleft lip. The syndrome occurs when pharyngeal pouches 3 and 4 fail to differentiate into the thymus and the parathyroid glands. In addition, abnormal neural crest migration results in facial anomalies and cardiovascular anomalies involving the aorticopulmonary (AP) septum.

49–E. Individuals with testicular feminization syndrome lack ovaries. The most common cause of testicular feminization syndrome is the lack of androgen receptors in the urethral folds and genital swellings of the embryo. Therefore, the individual develops female external genitalia; the 46,XY genotype directs the formation of testes.

50–A. The pleuropericardial membranes separate the pericardial cavity from the pleural cavity and develop into the fibrous pericardium surrounding the heart.

51–E. A foramen secundum defect, the most common clinically significant type of atrial septal defect (ASD), produces a patent foramen ovale, a large opening between the right and left atria. It is caused by excessive resorption of the septum primum or septum secundum.

52–H. Tricuspid atresia, a type of atrioventricular (AV) septal defect, is caused by obliteration of the right AV canal. It is always marked by patent foramen ovale, interventricular (IV) septal defect, overdeveloped left ventricle, and underdeveloped right ventricle.

53–D. Transposition of the great arteries is a type of aorticopulmonary (AP) septal defect. It is caused by abnormal neural crest cell migration, which results in failure of the AP septum to form in a spiral fashion.

54–A. Tetralogy of Fallot–pulmonary stenosis, overriding aorta, interventricular (IV) septal defect, and right ventricular hypertrophy–is a type of aorticopulmonary (AP) septal defect. It is caused by a failure of the openings of the pulmonary trunk and aorta to align with the openings of the ventricles.

55–B. The most common congenital cardiac malformation is a ventricular septal defect (VSD). Of the VSDs, membranous VSD is the most common type.

56–C. Persistent truncus arteriosus is a type of aorticopulmonary (AP) septal defect. Abnormal neural crest cell migration results in the incomplete formation of the AP septum.

57–F. The cause of coarctation of the aorta, in which the lumen of the artery is constricted, is unclear. There are two types: postductal coarctation, which occurs inferior to the ductus arteriosus and is the most common type, and preductal coarctation, which occurs superior to the ductus arteriosus.

58–G. The ductus arteriosus is the connection between the pulmonary artery and aorta. It normally closes soon after birth to form the ligamentum arteriosum in the adult.

59–J. CN X innervates the structures of pharyngeal arches 4 and 6, including the constrictors of the pharynx and the intrinsic muscles of the larynx.

60–C. CN III is derived from the basal plate of the rostral midbrain. It receives general somatic efferent (GSE) fibers from the oculomotor nucleus and general visceral efferent (GVE) fibers from the Edinger-Westphal nucleus.

61–E. CN V innervates the structures of pharyngeal arch 1.

62–B. CN II is derived from the diencephalon; it is a pathway (tract) of the CNS.

63–I. CN IX innervates the structures of pharyngeal arch 3.

64–L. CN XII arises from the hypoglossal nucleus, the only GSE nucleus found in the medulla.

65–D. CN IV is derived from the basal plate of the caudal midbrain; it is the only cranial nerve that completely decussates within the brain stem, and exits from the dorsal surface of the midbrain.

66–G. CN VII innervates the structures of pharyngeal arch 2.

67–F. CN VI arises from the abducent nucleus, the only GSE nucleus of the pons; it innervates one muscle, the lateral rectus.

68–H. CN VIII is derived from the otic placode.

69–L. CN XII innervates the intrinsic and extrinsic muscles of the tongue, which are derivatives of the occipital somites. Palatoglossus muscle is the exception and is innervated by CN X.

70–C. CN III innervates extraocular muscles derived from the preotic myotomes (somites), and the sphincter pupillae muscle of the iris is derived from the neuroectoderm.

71–E. Hydranencephaly usually presents as huge intracerebral cavitation resulting from in utero infarction in the territory of the internal carotid artery. Hydranencephaly may be caused by in utero infection with *Toxoplasma*, rubella, cytomegalovirus, herpesvirus, or other viruses (mnemonic = TORCH).

72–D. Holoprosencephaly, which is commonly seen in trisomy 13 (Patau syndrome) and has been reported in fetal alcohol syndrome, is characterized by a single ventricular cavity and agenesis of the olfactory bulbs and tracts (arhinencephaly).

73–D. Holoprosencephaly is characterized by a single ventricular cavity and agenesis of the olfactory bulbs and tracts (arhinencephaly). Holoprosencephaly results from failure of midline cleavage of the embryonic forebrain.

74–A. Failure of the anterior neuropore to close results in anencephaly.

75–C. Dandy-Walker syndrome results from atresia of the outlet foramina of the fourth ventricle; it develops at the end of the first trimester when the foramina of Luschka and Magendie fail to perforate.

76–B. Arnold-Chiari malformation is characterized by herniation of caudal vermis and cerebellar tonsils through the foramen magnum.

77–E. The basilar membrane separates the cochlear duct from the scala tympani.

78–D. The tectorial membrane is found in the cochlear duct, an endolymphatic space. The tectorial membrane is a glycoproteinaceous substance secreted by the interdental cells of the spiral limbus. The microvilli of the hair cells are embedded in the membrane.

79–B. The iridopupillary membrane consists of vascular mesodermal tissue, which covers the pupil. This membrane is usually resorbed before birth. It may be seen after birth as the persistent iridopupillary membrane.

80–D. The microvilli (stereocilia) of the hair cells of the organ of Corti are embedded in the tectorial membrane.

81–C. The tympanic membrane is derived from the three germ layers (ectoderm, mesoderm, and endoderm) associated with pharyngeal membrane 1.

82–D. The bony modiolus contains the spiral ganglion of the cochlear nerve, which contains bipolar neurons.

83–A. The basilar membrane, which lies between the scala tympani and the scala media (cochlear duct), has pitch localization; high tones (20,000 Hz) are perceived at its base and low tones (20 Hz) at its apex.

84–E. The scala tympani (and scala vestibuli) contains perilymph, which communicates with the subarachnoid space of the posterior cranial fossa via the perilymphatic duct (cochlear aqueduct).

85–C. The vestibular membrane (Reissner's membrane) separates the scala vestibuli from the cochlear duct (scala media).

86–B. The cochlear duct contains endolymph, which is produced by the stria vascularis.

87–B. The dilator and sphincter muscles of the iris are derived from the neuroectoderm of the optic cup.

88–C. Aqueous humor is produced by the epithelial lining of the ciliary processes of the ciliary body.

89–D. The vitreous body is formed from mesodermal cells that migrate through the choroid (optic) fissure, forming a transparent gelatinous substance between the lens and retina.

90–E. The hyaloid canal (Cloquet's canal) is a remnant of the hyaloid artery, a branch of the ophthalmic artery that irrigates the developing lens and retina during the embryonic and early fetal periods. Occasionally a vestige of the hyaloid artery can be seen with the ophthalmoscope.

91–A. The lens develops from the lens placode, which derives from the surface ectoderm.

92–A. "A" points to the utricle, which contains the macula utriculi. The utricle is derived from the utricular division of the otic vesicle; the utricular division of the otic vesicle also gives rise to the semicircular ducts and the endolymphatic sac and duct.

93–E. High-pitched sounds are localized in the base of the cochlea; low-pitched sounds are localized in its apex.

94–B. "B" points to the saccule of the membranous labyrinth. The saccular division of the otic vesicle gives rise to the saccule and the cochlear duct. The ductus reuniens interconnects the saccule and the scala media (cochlear duct).

95–F. The endolymphatic sac is thought to be the site of endolymph absorption.

96–G. Within the ampulla of a semicircular duct lies the crista ampullaris and its sensory (hair) cells, which respond to angular acceleration (flow of endolymph).

97–B. "B" points to the saccule of the membranous labyrinth, which contains the macula sacculi.

98–I. Because of abnormal neural crest migration, no parasympathetic ganglion cells are found in certain areas of the large intestine in Hirschsprung disease.

99–A. If the tracheoesophageal septum deviates too far dorsally, the esophagus will end as a blind tube.

100–E. The U-shaped midgut (midgut loop) herniates into the extraembryonic coelom (physiological umbilical herniation) beginning at week 6 and is reduced by week 11. If the intestines fail to return to the abdominal cavity, an omphalocele forms.

101–H. The midgut normally undergoes a 270° counterclockwise rotation. If only a partial rotation occurs, a twisting of the intestines (volvulus) may occur; this may obstruct passage of intestinal contents or may produce necrosis because of compromised blood supply.

102–D. Accelerated development of pancreatic islets is associated with increased birth weight. It occurs when fetal islets are exposed to high levels of glucose, such as those present in a pregnancy involving a diabetic woman. The increased fetal insulin levels cause fat and glycogen deposition in fetal tissues.

103–F. If the vitelline duct persists, an ileal diverticulum will occur. The outpouching may connect to the umbilicus via a fibrous cord or fistula.

104–B. Hypertrophic pyloric stenosis occurs when the muscle layer in the pyloric region hypertrophies, causing a narrow pyloric lumen that obstructs food passage. It is clinically associated with projectile vomiting and palpation of a small knot at the right costal margin.

105–G. Gastroschisis occurs when the muscle and integumentary layers fail to form completely, resulting in protrusion of abdominal viscera.

106–C. During development, the endodermal lining of the gallbladder and extrahepatic bile ducts proliferates and obliterates the lumen. Later, recanalization occurs. Extrahepatic biliary atresia is associated clinically with jaundice soon after birth, white clay-colored stool, and dark-colored urine.

107–J. If abnormal formation of the urorectal septum occurs, the anal canal may end as a blind sac below the puborectalis muscle. Anal agenesis is usually associated with rectovesical fistula, rectourethral fistula, or rectovaginal fistula.

108–K. Anorectal agenesis occurs when the rectum ends as a blind sac above the puborectalis muscle due to abnormal formation of the urorectal septum. It is the most common type of anorectal malformation.

109–E. The recurrent laryngeal branch of the vagus nerve (CN X) is the nerve of pharyngeal arch 6; it innervates the intrinsic muscles of the larynx.

110–D. The superior laryngeal branch of the vagus nerve (CN X) is the nerve of pharyngeal arch 4; it innervates all skeletal muscles of the soft palate except the tensor veli palatini, which is innervated by CN V, and all skeletal muscles of the pharynx except the stylopharyngeus, which is innervated by CN IX.

111–B. The muscles of facial expression are innervated by the facial nerve, the nerve of pharyngeal arch 2.

112–A. The muscles of mastication are innervated by the trigeminal nerve (CN V), the nerve of pharyngeal arch 1.

113–D. The constrictor muscles of the pharynx are innervated by the superior laryngeal branch of the vagus nerve (CN X); the superior laryngeal nerve is the nerve of pharyngeal arch 4.

114–B. Infants with microcephaly have small brains (micrencephaly) and are mentally retarded.

115–B. Microcephaly is seen frequently as the result of an in utero infection with rubella virus, cytomegalovirus, or *Toxoplasma gondii.*

116–A. Acromegaly is characterized by large jaw, hands, and feet; it is the result of an excessive elaboration of growth hormone (hyperpituitarism).

117–E. Scaphocephaly is characterized by a long skull, which results from premature closure of the sagittal suture.

118–C. Oxycephaly (turricephaly or acrocephaly) is a towerlike skull resulting from premature closure of the lambdoid and coronal sutures.

119–D. Cementum is formed by cementoblasts derived from the inner cells of the dental sac and is found between the dentin and the periodontal ligament.

120–B. The dental papilla, derived from the neural crest, gives rise to the odontoblasts, which produce dentin.

121–A. Ameloblasts develop from the enamel organ and produce enamel.

122–B. Odontoblasts, derived from the dental papilla (of neural crest origin), produce dentin.

123–A. Ameloblasts are derived from ectoderm.

124–D. The use of diazepam, an anxiolytic, in the first trimester has resulted in craniofacial deformities.

125–G. The antibiotic streptomycin is known to cause sensorineural deafness.

126–F. Retinoic acid, used to treat chronic dermatoses, is a known teratogen shown to cause neural tube defects (spina bifida cystica) and cardiovascular anomalies.

127–H. The maternal serum level of unconjugated estriol is reduced when the fetus has Down syndrome; it is also reduced in cases of fetal immaturity and in women who are smokers.

128–A. Low maternal alpha-fetoprotein serum levels are associated with Down syndrome (trisomy 21).

129–A. High maternal serum values of alpha-fetoprotein are associated with neural tube defects, such as spina bifida, and anencephaly.

130–B. The use of aminopterin, a folic acid antagonist, during pregnancy has resulted in intrauterine growth retardation, anencephaly, spina bifida, hydrocephalus, and cleft lip and palate.

131–E. Use of potassium iodide during pregnancy has resulted in thyroid hyperplasia and mental retardation (cretinism).

132–C. The brains of older patients with Down syndrome have the neuropathology of Alzheimer disease (i.e., neuritic plaques, neurofibrillary tangles, amyloid deposition, and granulovacuolar degeneration). Nervous system amyloid protein is coded in chromosome 21.

133–E. The use of oral contraceptives (progestogens and estrogens) during pregnancy may result in the VACTERL syndrome, consisting of Vertebral, Anal, Cardiac, Tracheoesophageal, Renal, and Limb malformations.

134–B. DiGeorge syndrome is characterized by an absence of the thymus and parathyroid glands and T-cell insufficiency.

135–D. Prader-Willi syndrome is associated with a chromosome deletion of band q12 on chromosome 15 found in the father.

136–A. Angelman syndrome is associated with a chromosome deletion of band q12 on chromosome 15 found in the mother.

Index

Page numbers followed by f refer to figures; page numbers followed by t refer to tables.

A

Abducens nerve, 94
Accessory nerve, 94
Accessory pancreatic duct, 130
Accessory ribs, 208
Achondroplasia, 210, 259
   paternal age and, 6
Acrocephaly, 203
Acromegaly, 210
Acrosome reaction, 13
Aeration, at birth, 143
AFP (alpha-fetoprotein), 74
AFP (alpha-fetoprotein) assay, 249
Afterbirth. See Placenta
Age, parental, and chromosomal ab-
   normalities, 6
Alar plate
   in mesencephalon development, 89,
      89f
   in metencephalon development, 88,
      88f
   in myelencephalon development,
      86f, 87
   in spinal cord development, 84
Albinism, 194
Alcohol abuse, and fetal development,
   263
Allantois, 68
Allocortex, development of, 92
Alopecia, 195
Alpha-fetoprotein (AFP), 74
Alpha-fetoprotein (AFP) assay, 249
Alveolar period, of lung development,
   142f, 143
Alzheimer's disease, genetic basis of,
   260
Amelia, 209
Aminopterin, and fetal development,
   262
Amniocentesis, 249, 250t
Amniochorionic membranes, prema-
   ture rupture of, 72
Amniotic band syndrome, 72
Amniotic fluid, 71-72
Ampulla of Vater, 130
Anal canal, development of, 134f, 134-
   135
Androgen, complete insensitivity to,
   188
Anencephaly, 96
Angelman syndrome, 259
Angiogenesis, 32-33
Ankyloglossia, 157
Annular pancreas, 130
Annulus fibrosus, 206
Anophthalmia, 118
Anorectal agenesis, 135

Antbiotics, and fetal development,
   262-263
Anterior condensation
   in lower limb development, 231,
      232f
   in upper limb development, 221,
      222f
Antigens, oncofetal, 23-24
Antimetabolites, and fetal develop-
   ment, 262
Antineoplastic agents, and fetal devel-
   opment, 262
Anus
   agenesis of, 135
   imperforate, 135
Aorta, coarctation of, postductal, 55,
   55f
Aortic arches, 54, 54t
   defects of, 55
Aorticopulmonary (AP) septum
   defects of, 48, 49f, 50
   formation of, 43-44, 46f
Aortic valve stenosis, 49f, 50
Apical ectodermal ridge, 217, 227
Aplasia, 257
Appendix, development of, 131, 131f
AP septum. See Aorticopulmonary
   (AP) septum
Aqueductal stenosis, 98
Aqueous humor, 115
Arhinencephaly, 99, 99f
Arnold-Chiari malformation, 96, 97f
Arteries. See also specific names
   development of, 54t, 54-56, 55f
Astroglia, formation of, 83
Atlas, 204
Atrial septal defects, 50f, 50-51
Atrial septum, formation of, 44, 46f
Atrioventricular (AV) canal, common,
   persistent, 51, 52f
Atrioventricular (AV) septal defect,
   51, 52f, 53
Atrioventricular (AV) septum, forma-
   tion of, 44-45, 47f
Atrium, common, 50f, 50-51
Auditory meatus, external
   atresia of, 109
   development of, 108
Auricle
   development of, 108
   malformation of, 109
Autonomic nervous system, develop-
   ment of, 93, 93f
Autosomal abnormalities, 258
AV (atrioventricular) septal defect,
   51, 52f, 53
AV (atrioventricular) septum, forma-
   tion of, 44-45, 47f
Axillary artery, 218f

Axis, 204
Axis artery, 218f, 219, 229

B

Barr bodies, 3
Basal plate
   in mesencephalon development, 89f,
      89-90
   in metencephalon development, 88,
      88f
   in myelencephalon development,
      86f, 87
   in spinal cord development, 84
Basis pedunculi, 90
Bicornuate uterus, 179, 179f
Bile ducts, extrahepatic, development
   of, 128f, 128-129
Biliary atresia, extrahepatic, 128
Biopsy, chorionic villus, 249-250, 250t
Bipartite placenta, 72
Birth
   aeration of lungs at, 143
   circulatory changes at, 71
Birth defects, 257-265
   classification of, 257
   drugs and, 262-264
   failure of neural crest cell migra-
      tion and, 265
   genetic factors in, 257-260
      numerical chromosomal abnormal-
         ities, 257-259
      structural chromosomal abnormal-
         ities, 259-260
   infectious agents and, 260-261
   maternal hyperthermia and, 265
   multifactorial, 260
   parity and, 264
   radiation and, 264
   substance abuse and, 263-264
Bladder
   development of, 166-167, 167f
   exstrophy of, 170
Blastocyst, formation of, 15
Blastocyte, formation of, 14f, 14-15
Block vertebra, 207f, 208
Body cavities, formation of, 237-240
   intraembryonic coelom, 237f-239f,
      237-239
Bone, formation of
   in lower limbs, 229, 230f
   in upper limbs, 219, 220f
Bony labyrinth, 105f-106f, 107-108
Brachial plexus, 218f
   development of, 222f, 222-223
Brain. See also Nervous system
   embryologic zones of, 84
   vesicles of, development of, 81-82,
      82f, 83t